T0093609

RevMED

300 SBAs in
Clinical Specialties

Other Related Titles from World Scientific

RevMED 300 SBAs in Medicine and Surgery
by Lasith Ranasinghe and Oliver Clements
ISBN: 978-1-78634-681-0
ISBN: 978-1-78634-711-4 (pbk)

300 Single Best Answers in Clinical Medicine
by George Collins, James Davis and Oscar Swift
edited by Huw Beynon
ISBN: 978-1-78326-436-0
ISBN: 978-1-78326-437-7 (pbk)

320 Single Best Answer Questions for Final Year Medical Students
Second Edition
by Adam Ioannou
ISBN: 978-981-121-008-2
ISBN: 978-981-121-077-8 (pbk)

The PICU Book: A Primer for Medical Students, Residents and Acute Care Practitioners
edited by Ronald M Perkin, Irma Fiordalisi and William E Novotny
ISBN: 978-981-4329-60-6

Surgical Talk: Lecture Notes in Undergraduate Surgery
Third Edition
by Andrew Goldberg and Gerard Stansby
ISBN: 978-1-84816-614-1 (pbk)

RevMED

300 SBAs in
Clinical Specialties

Lasith Ranasinghe • Oliver Clements

Imperial College London, UK

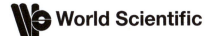

World Scientific

EW JERSEY · LONDON · SINGAPORE · BEIJING · SHANGHAI · HONG KONG · TAIPEI · CHENNAI · TOKYO

Published by

World Scientific Publishing Europe Ltd.
57 Shelton Street, Covent Garden, London WC2H 9HE
Head office: 5 Toh Tuck Link, Singapore 596224
USA office: 27 Warren Street, Suite 401-402, Hackensack, NJ 07601

Library of Congress Control Number: 2020007592

British Library Cataloguing-in-Publication Data
A catalogue record for this book is available from the British Library.

REVMED 300 SBAS IN CLINICAL SPECIALTIES

ISBN 978-1-78634-846-3 (hardcover)
ISBN 978-1-78634-852-4 (paperback)
ISBN 978-1-78634-847-0 (ebook for Institutions)
ISBN 978-1-78634-848-7 (ebook for Individuals)

For any available supplementary material, please visit
https://www.worldscientific.com/worldscibooks/10.1142/Q0250#t=suppl

Desk Editors: Aanand Jayaraman/Michael Beale/Shi Ying Koe

Typeset by Stallion Press
Email: enquiries@stallionpress.com

*To my parents, my brother and my sister-in-law for supporting
me through thick and thin. To the amazing community
at Imperial College School of Medicine for giving me the
best years of my life and, finally, to my niece,
Ayana, for inspiring me to be my best self.*

—Lasith Ranasinghe

*To Ros, my mum, my dad and my brothers,
Matt, Alex and Chris, for your love, encouragement
and continuous support throughout medical school
and to the boys at ICSM for an unforgettable six years.*

—Oliver Clements

Foreword

It has always been interesting to me that the beginning of the Hippocratic oath, written between the 5th and the 3rd century BC, is so little known. The oldest written version is held in the Vatican library and dates back to the 10th century. The first paragraph of importance speaks of the relationship between teachers and their students. It uses the language of family to describe the bond that can develop between people who are learning together.

It is in the context of this ancient promise that I am delighted to write the Foreword for this excellent book of SBAs. Lasith and Oliver have always been fascinated by education and through this book they are expanding the reach of their teaching prowess from the small(ish) family of Imperial College to the wider world, in keeping with the Hippocratic tradition. Their old teachers are very proud of them and I for one am sure that the people that use this book will understand why.

Mr. Martin Lupton
Vice Dean (Education)
Head of Undergraduate School of Medicine
Imperial College School of Medicine

Preface

Preparing for exams in the clinical specialties can be difficult because, although the general principles of anatomy, physiology, and pharmacology remain relevant, the three specialties tend to occupy their own niche in the medical curriculum with many concepts that would not have been encountered when studying general medicine and surgery. Furthermore, the sensitive nature of the three clinical specialties means that it is important for students to follow evidence-based guidelines whilst maintaining a patient-centred approach and an awareness of the clinical and ethical responsibilities of doctors.

This book was written soon after we completed our exams in the clinical specialties which, we feel, were the toughest of our time at medical school. The ability to use your clinical acumen to subtly differentiate between differentials and formulate a management plan are essential to doing well in these exams. Although rote learning from textbooks may have its place in the build-up to exams, putting your knowledge to the test and learning through the use of worked examples in SBA books is a much more engaging and efficient way of learning the content. We encourage students, even if you are not confident in your current level of knowledge, to attempt the questions in this book and study the explanations as they are meticulously crafted to concisely convey the important information about a topic with visual aids such as management flowcharts. As this book is written by students and edited by registrars and consultants, we have combined a student-friendly and exam-focused delivery with clinical accuracy and real-life principles of treatment.

We hope that this will be useful in your revision and wish you all the best for your exams in clinical specialties!

About the Authors

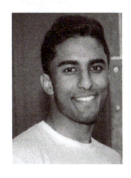

Lasith Ranasinghe is a final year Medical Student at Imperial College School of Medicine. He grew up in Norwich before starting Medicine at Imperial College London in 2014. He has developed an interest in medical education having delivered several lectures to younger students, co-chairing the Medical Education (MedED) society, and undertaking the role of Academic Officer on the Students' Union. He has maintained a high academic standard, consistently being placed in the top 10 in his cohort, and achieving 15 prizes for academic excellence. In his spare time, he runs two charities, 'Smile', which raises money to improve the standard of education for underprivileged children in Sri Lanka, and 'Make a Medic', which collects used medical educational resources in the UK and ships them to medical schools in developing countries. He also enjoys playing football and cricket for ICSM FC and IMCC, respectively. He will soon be starting an Academic Foundation Programme in Paediatrics with Imperial College London in the North West Thames deanery.

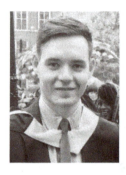

Oliver Clements is a final year Medical Student at Imperial College School of Medicine. Originally from High Wycombe, he was the only student from his secondary school to gain admission to medical school. During his time at Imperial College London, he has got involved with various educational initiatives, such as organising OSCE and PACES tutorials. He has maintained a high standard at medical school, having achieved merits in 1st and 2nd year, as well as merits in PACES and pathology and distinctions in obstetrics & gynaecology and psychiatry in 5th year. He has a First Class (Hons) in Gastroenterology and Hepatology and has published his exceptional research in cholangiocarcinoma in the *Journal of Hepatology* and presented his work at two international conferences. He was awarded Naranjan Singh Virdee prize for his research. In his spare time, he enjoys fitness and playing football.

List of Editors and Illustrators

EDITORS

Dr. Michael Malley — Paediatric Registrar (ST6) in Paediatric Emergency Medicine, Bristol Royal Hospital for Children.

Dr. Marie Monaghan — Paediatric Registrar (ST6), Bristol Royal Hospital for Children.

Dr. Ayesha Lodhia — Obstetrics & Gynaecology Registrar and Teaching Fellow, King's College Hospital NHS Foundation Trust.

Dr. Zoe Robinson — Obstetrics & Gynaecology Trainee, Severn Deanery.

Dr. Donna Arya — Consultant Forensic Psychiatrist, Elysium Healthcare.

ILLUSTRATOR

Yu Meng Li — Fifth Year Medical Student, Imperial College School of Medicine.

Acknowledgements

We would like to thank the staff at World Scientific Publishing for approaching this publication with such enthusiasm. We would also like to thank our editors and the younger medical students who helped design SBAs and explanations that conveyed expert-level content in a student-friendly manner. Finally, we would like to thank Imperial College School of Medicine for encouraging students to pursue ambitious projects and supporting us in our ventures.

Contents

Paediatrics: Paper 1

Questions

1. An 18-month-old girl is brought to A&E by her father. She has vomited several times over the last 24 hours. On examination, she is irritable and has a distended abdomen with tinkling bowel sounds. Which investigation is most likely to reveal the underlying diagnosis?

   A Abdominal ultrasound
   B Abdominal X-ray
   C Stool culture
   D Endoscopy
   E Faecal calprotectin

2. An 8-year-old boy is brought to see his GP as he has developed a rash on his face over the last 3 days. On inspection, the rash has a yellow, crusty appearance and is located in one discrete patch just below his mouth. What is the most appropriate treatment option?

   A Hygiene measures
   B Flucloxacillin
   C Clarithromycin
   D Aciclovir
   E Topical fusidic acid

3. A 3-year-old girl is brought to paediatric A&E after suffering from a severe cough. It started 2 days ago and tends to occur in abrupt bursts lasting a matter of minutes, which has once ended with her vomiting. She has had a cold and a runny nose for the past 1 week. On examination, a subconjunctival haemorrhage is noted. What is the most likely diagnosis?

   A Bronchiolitis
   B Whooping cough
   C Croup
   D Pneumonia
   E Acute epiglottitis

4. A 5-year-old boy with minimal change disease has recently had a relapse of nephrotic syndrome during which he became oedematous and required treatment with oral prednisolone. His parents have become concerned about the long-term complications of minimal change disease. Which of the following is a complication of minimal change disease?

   A Intracranial haemorrhage
   B Subarachnoid haemorrhage
   C Deep vein thrombosis
   D Chronic kidney disease
   E Urinary tract calculi

5. A neonate who underwent a traumatic delivery is unresponsive. After being dried with a towel, it is noted that he is floppy with a heart rate of 58 bpm and has not taken his first breath yet. What is the next step in his management?

   A Give 2 rescue breaths
   B Give 5 inflation breaths
   C Start chest compression
   D Intubate to secure the airway
   E Gain venous access

6. A 15-year-old girl has been experiencing pain in her right knee when she climbs stairs. She has not had any trauma to the area. She explains that she plays netball competitively and has to practise on most days. On examination, crepitus is palpable when the knee is extended, and she complains of a grating sensation. What is the most likely diagnosis?

    A Osgood–Schlatter disease
    B Chondromalacia patellae
    C Osteochondritis dissecans
    D Subluxation of the patella
    E Growing pains

7. A newborn girl, born 2 hours ago at 39 weeks' gestation, is found to be jaundiced on neonatal examination. She has a microcephaly and hepatosplenomegaly. Coombs' test is negative. What is the most likely cause of jaundice in this case?

    A Congenital infection
    B Physiological jaundice
    C Biliary atresia
    D Rhesus incompatibility
    E Congenital hypothyroidism

8. A 12-year-old girl has wet herself at school several times over the past few years. She also has a 3-year history of lower back pain that worsens with activity. On examination, power is reduced in both legs and a sacral dimple is observed. What is the most likely diagnosis?

    A Spina bifida occulta
    B Meningocele
    C Myelomeningocele
    D Anencephaly
    E Encephalocele

9. A 10-year-old boy with cystic fibrosis has developed a chronic cough productive of purulent sputum. It is suspected that he has developed

bronchiectasis. What is the best investigation to confirm a diagnosis of bronchiectasis?

   A Chest X-ray
   B Bronchoscopy
   C Spirometry
   D PET scan
   E CT scan

10. A 13-year-old boy is brought to A&E feeling lethargic and drowsy. He has had a bad episode of diarrhoea and vomiting for the past 3 days. On examination, he has dry mucous membranes, reduced skin turgor and mottled skin with a capillary refill time of 4 seconds. His observations are as follows:

Heart rate: 135 bpm
Blood pressure: 82/46 mm Hg
Respiratory rate: 27 breaths/min
Temperature: 37.2°C

What is the most appropriate initial management option?

   A Admit and give an intravenous bolus of 0.9% sodium chloride solution
   B Admit and start oral rehydration solution
   C Admit and start broad spectrum antibiotics
   D Discharge with a course of antibiotics
   E Discharge with a course of antibiotics and loperamide

11. A 1-day-old neonate has developed a swelling on his scalp that was not present at the time of birth. On examination, the neonate has a soft swelling over his right parietal bone which does not cross the suture lines. The child has been well since birth, however, was delivered with the assistance of a ventouse due to failure to progress through the second stage. What is the most likely diagnosis?

   A Cranial moulding
   B Caput succedaneum

C Cephalohaematoma

D Subgaleal haemorrhage

E Craniosynostosis

12. A 3-year-old boy is referred to a developmental clinic due to difficulties in walking. He has a waddling gait and bulky calves. His mum tells you that he is clumsy and falls over frequently and is unable to climb stairs without being helped. He did not walk unsupported until he was 20 months old, and did not know more than 6 words until he was 18 months old. What is the most likely underlying diagnosis?

   A Charcot–Marie–Tooth disease

   B Duchenne muscular dystrophy

   C Becker muscular dystrophy

   D Myotonic dystrophy

   E Spinal muscular atrophy

13. What is the most common cause of meningitis?

   A *Neisseria meningitidis*

   B *Haemophilus influenzae*

   C *Streptococcus pneumoniae*

   D Enteroviruses

   E Herpes simplex virus

14. A 2-month-old boy presents to clinic with his mother who claims that he turns blue and becomes short of breath during feeds. He has also been struggling to gain weight and has fallen by 5 centiles. On examination, there is an ejection systolic murmur at the left sternal edge. What is the most likely diagnosis?

   A Persistent ductus arteriosus

   B Tetralogy of Fallot

   C Transposition of the great arteries

   D Ventricular septal defect

   E Atrial septal defect

15. A 17-year-old boy is being reviewed in clinic. He is tall and slim with long, thin limbs. He is being monitored for an aortic aneurysm and cataracts. What is the inheritance pattern of the disorder being described?

    A Autosomal dominant
    B Autosomal recessive
    C X-linked recessive
    D X-linked dominant
    E Meiotic nondisjunction

16. A 3-year-old boy has been complaining of a pain in his left ear since the morning and has been more irritable than usual. On examination, his left tympanic membrane is bulging and cloudy with no discharge. His vital signs are as follows:

    Heart rate: 109 bpm
    Respiratory rate: 24 breaths/min
    Temperature: 38°C
    Blood pressure: 98/64 mm Hg

    What is the most appropriate management option?

    A Prescribe a 3-day course of amoxicillin
    B Prescribe a 7-day course of amoxicillin
    C Reassure and provide advice about pain relief
    D Admit to hospital for assessment
    E Refer to an ENT specialist

17. A 5-year-old Syrian boy is referred to paediatrics after his teacher commented that he runs differently from the other children. On examination, he has a waddling gait, his left leg is shorter than the right, there is limited abduction of the left hip and his skin folds are asymmetrical. Given the most likely diagnosis, what is the most appropriate 1st line investigation?

    A MRI
    B Plain X-ray
    C US scan

D CT scan
E No investigations required

18. A newborn boy, born 1 hour ago, has developed rapid, shallow breathing. On examination, there is marked chest recession, expiratory grunting, nasal flaring, and central cyanosis. He was born at 34 weeks' gestation to a mother with type 1 diabetes mellitus. A chest X-ray shows diffuse ground-glass shadowing with air bronchograms. What is the most likely diagnosis?

    A Transient tachypnoea of the newborn
    B Respiratory distress syndrome
    C Meconium aspiration
    D Persistent pulmonary hypertension of the newborn
    E Bronchopulmonary dysplasia

19. A 3-year-old boy is brought to see the GP as he has become constipated. He used to pass 1–2 stools per day but has not passed a stool in 7 days. The last stool he passed was dry and pellet-like. On examination, he complains of some abdominal discomfort and an indentable mass is palpated in his left iliac fossa. What is the most appropriate 1st line treatment option?

    A Senna
    B Polyethylene glycol and electrolytes
    C Lactulose enema
    D Advise on fluid intake and toileting techniques
    E Manual evacuation

20. A 10-month-old boy presents to clinic with asymmetric reaching and right-hand preference. On examination, there is increased tone in the left arm and leg with no abnormalities on the right side. Cerebral palsy is suspected. Which type of cerebral palsy is this most likely to be?

    A Spastic hemiplegic
    B Spastic quadriplegic

    C Spastic diplegic

    D Dyskinetic

    E Ataxic

21. An 11-year-old boy has developed a rash on his arms over the last
week. Initially, the rash appeared as pink blotches which have since
developed into well-defined target-shaped lesions. What is the most
likely underlying diagnosis?

    A Guttate psoriasis

    B Pityriasis versicolor

    C Erythema multiforme

    D Tinea corporis

    E Miliaria

22. A 6-month-old boy has been irritable with a runny nose over the past
two days. His mother adds that he has developed persistent dry cough
and his breathing has become noisy since this morning. On examination, a high-pitched expiratory wheeze can be auscultated throughout
the chest. He has continued to feed well. His vital signs are as follows:

Heart rate: 146 bpm
Respiratory rate: 42 breaths/min
Temperature: 37.2°C
Blood pressure: 86/54 mm Hg
Oxygen saturation: 97% on air

Which of the following is the most appropriate management option?

    A Reassure and discharge with a course of amoxicillin

    B Reassure and discharge with advice on conservative measures

    C Reassure and discharge with a course of palivizumab

    D Administer supplemental oxygen, give intravenous fluids, and
admit

    E Perform upper airways suctioning and admit

23. A 6-year-old girl has been unwell for the last week with abdominal
cramps, fever, and diarrhoea. Although her symptoms have improved,

she is now lethargic, looks pale with some bruising on her legs. She has also been urinating less frequently. What is the most likely underlying diagnosis?

A Thrombotic thrombocytopenic purpura
B Haemolytic uraemic syndrome
C Henoch–Schönlein purpura
D IgA nephropathy
E Post-streptococcal glomerulonephritis

24. A 17-year-old boy is worried that he has not started puberty yet. He is on the 99th centile for height and, on examination, he has gynaecomastia, a feminised physique and small testes. Which hormone profile is consistent with this presentation?

A Low FSH and LH and low testosterone
B Elevated FSH and LH and elevated testosterone
C Elevated FSH and LH and low testosterone
D Low FSH and LH and elevated testosterone
E Elevated TSH and low T4

25. The mother of an 8-year-old boy has come to discuss the influenza vaccine. He has moderate asthma which is currently being treated with inhaled beclomethasone and salbutamol. He has an allergy to egg that causes a hives-like rash. What is the most appropriate management option?

A Do not give the influenza vaccine
B Administer the IM influenza vaccine in the GP practice
C Administer the IM influenza vaccine in hospital
D Administer the nasal influenza vaccine in hospital
E Administer the IM influenza vaccine with IM adrenaline prophylaxis

26. A 4-year-old boy has been having several episodes of watery stools every day. His mother says that she often seen carrots and sweetcorn

mixed in with the stool but there is no blood or mucus. He denies experiencing any abdominal pain. Abdominal examination reveals no abnormalities. What is the most likely diagnosis?

A Toddler's diarrhoea
B Cow's milk protein allergy
C Coeliac disease
D Rotavirus infection
E Infantile colic

27. A 1-day-old neonate on the postnatal ward has become hypotonic with marked central cyanosis. His vital signs are as follows:

Temperature: 37.1°C
Blood pressure: 66/34 mm Hg
Heart rate: 156 bpm
Respiratory rate: 48 breaths/min
SaO_2: 82% on 85% oxygen via a non-rebreather mask

What is the most appropriate initial management?

A IV fluids
B IV benzylpenicillin and gentamicin
C IV alprostadil
D Emergency surgery
E Chest X-ray

28. A 4-year-old boy with autism and attention deficit hyperactivity disorder is being reviewed in clinic. On examination, he has a long face, large ears and large testicles. A pansystolic murmur can be auscultated. What is the most likely underlying diagnosis?

A William's syndrome
B Prader–Willi syndrome
C Noonan syndrome
D Fragile X syndrome
E DiGeorge syndrome

29. A 3-year-old boy has become increasingly constipated over the past 2 months. He has also lost weight, dropping from the 50th centile to the 20th centile in this time. On examination, a large abdominal mass is palpable, there is some bruising under his eyes and weakness in his legs. A neuroblastoma is suspected. Which of the following findings would support this diagnosis?

    A A loss of the red reflex on ophthalmoscopy
    B The presence of Reed–Sternberg cells on bone marrow biopsy
    C The presence of >20% lymphoblasts on bone marrow biopsy
    D Raised catecholamine metabolite levels on urine quantification
    E Periosteal reaction in radiographs

30. A 2-month old baby boy is brought into A&E with two bruises on his right arm. His mother reports that he rolled off the table while she was trying to change his nappy. On examination, the child appears distressed when his right arm is palpated, but the Moro reflex is present and the humerus does not appear fractured. What is the most appropriate first step in the management of this patient?

    A Admit to the paediatric ward
    B Refer for X-ray of affected arm
    C Refer for MRI of affected arm
    D Take bloods for coagulation screen
    E Urgently refer to paediatric orthopaedics

Answers

1. A

Intussusception is a condition that mainly occurs in young children (<2 years) and is characterised by telescoping of a section of the intestines. It most commonly occurs at the ileocaecal junction. Patients can present with features of bowel obstruction (vomiting, absolute constipation, abdominal distention) or they may describe an intermittent course where the child becomes irritable, pale and draws their legs up to their chest. Blood-stained 'redcurrant jelly stools' are classically associated with intussusception, however, this is a late sign that requires urgent intervention. Intussusception may develop after a non-specific febrile illness. This is thought to be due to enlarged Peyer's patches acting as a lead point for the intussusception. An abdominal ultrasound scan focusing on the affected part of the intestines may reveal 'target sign'. An abdominal X-ray may be useful to demonstrate bowel obstruction, however, it would not necessarily reveal the underlying diagnosis. Intussusception is usually treated using rectal air insufflation with fluoroscopy guidance. This involves pumping air into the intestines to reverse the intussusception. Occasionally, if this is unsuccessful, a surgical approach will be necessary. Patients should also be nil-by-mouth, have a nasogastric tube inserted and given adequate fluid resuscitation. Recurrent intussusception may warrant further investigation to search for a pathological lead point (e.g. Meckel's diverticulum).

2. E

This patient has developed impetigo — a common skin infection caused by *Staphylococcus aureus* or *Streptococcus pneumoniae*. It is often described as having a golden-yellow, crusted appearance. Hygiene measures should be recommended (e.g. hand washing after touching the lesions) to all patients. The 1st line treatment for localised disease is topical fusidic acid. More extensive disease will be treated using oral flucloxacillin. Clarithromycin is an alternative that can be used in penicillin-allergic patients. School exclusion should be advised until the lesions have crusted over. Impetigo usually heals without causing any skin scarring. Aciclovir is an antiviral agent that is mainly used to treat herpes simplex virus infections.

3. B

Whooping cough is a respiratory tract infection that is caused by *Bordatella pertussis*. It is becoming less common in developed countries since its introduction to the childhood vaccination schedule. It tends to initially cause a week of coryzal symptoms (known as the catarrhal phase) followed by the development of paroxysmal bouts of coughing. They are typically worse at night and may be severe enough to cause vomiting. Gasping for air between coughs may give rise to the characteristic 'whoop' that gives the disease its name. Vigorous coughing can lead to nosebleeds and subconjunctival haemorrhages. Patients may experience bouts of coughing for up to 3 months. If patients are diagnosed within 21 days of the onset of symptoms, they may benefit from a macrolide antibiotic (e.g. azithromycin). As it is a highly contagious disease, parents should be advised to keep children away from school/nursery until 48 hours of antibiotics have been completed or until 21 days after the onset of symptoms.

Bronchiolitis tends to follow a mild, self-limiting course with coryzal symptoms and a wheeze. Furthermore, the vast majority of cases occur in patients under the age of 1 year. Croup presents with a barking cough and stridor. Pneumonia will cause a cough, fever, and increased respiratory rate. Acute epiglottitis is a potentially life-threatening condition in which there is a rapid swelling of the epiglottis caused by *Haemophilus influenzae* type b. Children will typically present acutely unwell with a high fever and a painful throat that limits their ability to speak or swallow. There may be a soft stridor and the child may be sitting upright, immobile, and drooling from the mouth. Fortunately, acute epiglottitis has become very rare after the introduction of the *Haemophilus influenzae* type b vaccine.

4. C

Minimal change disease is the most common cause of nephrotic syndrome in children. Nephrotic syndrome presents with a triad of proteinuria, hypoalbuminaemia, and oedema. Although it usually responds to steroids, some patients will experience relapses and may develop complications. There are three main complications of minimal change disease: increased risk of thrombosis, increased risk of infection, and hypercholesterolaemia.

The loss of anti-thrombin III in the urine leads to a hypercoagulable state which may be further exacerbated by the thrombocytosis that is caused by steroid therapy. This can increase the risk of both venous thrombosis (e.g. deep vein thrombosis) and arterial thrombosis (e.g. myocardial infarction). The loss of immunoglobulins in the urine will increase the risk of infection, particularly by encapsulated bacteria (e.g. *Streptococcus pneumoniae*) so patients should receive appropriate vaccinations. The falling oncotic pressure due to urinary albumin losses is thought to trigger increased hepatic cholesterol synthesis resulting in hypercholesterolaemia. This will increase their cardiovascular risk.

Although minimal change disease affects the kidneys, it is rarely associated with chronic kidney disease or urinary tract calculi. Subarachnoid haemorrhage resulting from berry aneurysm rupture is associated with polycystic kidney disease. Furthermore, the hypercoagulable state in minimal change disease increases a patient's risk of thrombosis rather than haemorrhage.

5. B

Neonatal resuscitation follows a step-by-step process listed in the following. It is worth noting that 'inflation breaths' are the preferred term in neonatal resuscitation as it is designed to inflate the lungs and promote the clearance of fluid from the lungs. These breaths are slower and more prolonged than 'rescue breaths' used in basic life support. The neonatal resuscitation protocol differs from adult resuscitation protocols as it focuses mainly on respiratory as opposed to cardiac resuscitation. This is because the main cause of the bradycardia in neonates is hypoxia.

1. Dry the baby
2. Assess tone, breathing rate, and heart rate
3. If gasping or not breathing → give 5 inflation breaths
4. Reassess
5. If chest is not moving → consider 2-person airway control and repeat inflation breaths
6. If chest is moving but heart rate is <60 bpm → ventilate for 30 seconds

7. Reassess → if heart rate <60 bpm → start chest compressions with ventilation breaths (3:1)
8. Reassess every 30 seconds
9. If heart rate remains <60 bpm → consider venous access and drugs (e.g. atropine)

6. B

Chondromalacia patellae is defined as anterior knee pain caused by degeneration of the articular cartilage on the posterior surface of the patella. It is particularly common in young adults as a result of overuse in physical activities. The pain may be exacerbated by running, climbing stairs, and getting up from a chair. Passive movements are usually pain-less, but repeated extension may produce pain and a grating feeling, and crepitus or a small effusion may be palpable. Patients should receive physiotherapy to strengthen the quadriceps.

Osgood–Schlatter disease is the inflammation of the insertion of the patella ligament into the tibial tuberosity. It typically affects physically active adolescent boys and presents with knee pain following exercise with localised tenderness and swelling over the tibial tuberosity. Osteochondritis dissecans is a condition in which cracks form in the articular cartilage and subchondral bone, caused by reduced blood flow. Ensuing avascular necrosis results in fragmentation of the bone and carti-lage and free movement of these fragments within the joint space leads to activity-related pain, catching, locking, and giving way. Subluxation of the patellar is partial dislocation of the patella that produces a feeling of instability or giving way of the knee and, rarely, patellar dislocation. Growing pains are episodes of generalised aching in the legs that is sym-metrical, worst at night, and never present at the start of the day with no limitation of physical activities and no abnormalities on examination.

7. A

Jaundice in the first 24 hours of life is always pathological and infants should have their serum bilirubin measured urgently (within 2 hours) and then every 6 hours until the level is below the treatment threshold and stable or falling. The causes of neonatal jaundice can be divided according to the age of the infant.

<24 hours	24 hours–2 weeks	>2 weeks
Haemolytic disorders: rhesus incompatibility, ABO incompatibility, glucose-6-phosphate dehydrogenase deficiency, pyruvate kinase deficiency, hereditary spherocytosis	Physiological or breast milk jaundice Bruising (from instrumental delivery) Infection (e.g. UTI) Haemolytic disorders Polycythaemia Crigler Najjar syndrome	Bile duct obstruction (e.g. biliary atresia) Physiological or breast milk jaundice Infection Congenital hypothyroidism Haemolytic disorders High gastrointestinal obstruction (e.g. pyloric stenosis)
Congenital infection		Neonatal hepatitis

Physiological jaundice is very common in neonates due to the increased rate of red cell haemolysis and immature hepatic function. This usually starts after 24 hours of life and settles by 14 days. Biliary atresia is the abnormal development of the bile ducts which presents with jaundice after 2 weeks with pale stools, dark urine and failure to gain weight. Congenital hypothyroidism presents with excessive sleepiness, hypotonia, constipation, poor feeding, jaundice, and may have signs such as an umbilical hernia and macroglossia. Rhesus incompatibility is rare in the UK due to the use of anti-D immunoglobulin. It causes haemolytic disease, so Coombs' test would be positive. The congenital infections can be remembered using the mnemonic **TORCH** (**T**oxoplasmosis, **O**ther e.g. syphilis, **R**ubella, **C**ytomegalovirus, and **H**erpes simplex virus). Features common to all the TORCH infections include prematurity, jaundice, microcephaly, hepatosplenomegaly, thrombocytopenia, anaemia, and seizures. The infant in this case is demonstrating some of these features, making congenital infection the most likely answer.

8. A

Spina bifida occulta is a neural tube defect that occurs due to failure of fusion of the vertebral arch. It is often an incidental finding on X-ray, but there may be an overlying skin lesion, such as a tuft of hair, lipoma, birth mark, or dermal sinus. Tethered spinal cord syndrome is a complication of spina bifida occulta that describes fixation of the inelastic tissue of the caudal spine which causes abnormal movement of the spinal cord as the child grows. Disease progression is highly variable, but most develop an insidious onset of symptoms in childhood. Symptoms include lower back pain that worsens with activity, gait disturbance, scoliosis, high-arched feet, and neurological dysfunction (e.g. numbness or weakness, bladder and bowel dysfunction). Surgery is required to untether the spinal cord.

Meningocele and myelomeningocele are the two other forms of spina bifida. Meningocele describes herniation of the meninges between the vertebrae forming a sac that contains cerebrospinal fluid. Neurology is normal since the sac does not contain neural tissue, but the sac is at risk of rupture, causing meningitis and hydrocephalus. Myelomeningocele is the most severe form of spina bifida and occurs when the spinal cord is able to protrude through an opening in an unfused portion of the spinal column. It is associated with severe neurological complications such as paresis, talipes, neuropathic bowel and bladder, and hydrocephalus. Anencephaly is the failure of development of most of the cranium and brain. Affected infants are usually stillborn or die shortly after birth. Encephalocele is herniation of the brain and meninges through a midline skull defect.

9. E

Bronchiectasis is defined as the permanent dilatation of the bronchi resulting in chronic shortness of breath productive of copious volumes of purulent sputum. It typically results from chronic lung inflammation leading to fibrosis and permanent dilatation of the bronchi. Causes include cystic fibrosis, post-infectious (e.g. whooping cough), and obstruction due to the presence of a foreign body. A CT scan is the best investigation to confirm the diagnosis of bronchiectasis. Bronchoscopy may be used if obstruction due to the presence of foreign body is the suspected cause. Management of bronchiectasis is complex, but may include the use of mucolytic agents, bronchodilators, and prophylactic antibiotics. In severe cases, lung transplantation or resection of the bronchiectatic areas may be considered.

10. A

Dehydration is a serious complication of gastroenteritis which can lead to shock if fluid is not adequately replaced. Features of shock include mottled skin, cold extremities, delayed capillary refill, tachycardia, tachypnoea, and hypotension. This patient should be admitted and given an IV fluid bolus of 20 ml/kg of 0.9% sodium chloride solution. If the child remains shocked after the first bolus, a second bolus can be given. If larger fluid boluses are required, the patient should be transferred to HDU or PICU. Once the shock resolves, the child should be rehydrated with 0.9% sodium chloride and 5% dextrose. Maintenance fluids (daily requirements) are calculated based on weight as follows:

- 100 mL/kg/day for the first 10 kg of weight
- 50 mL/kg/day for the second 10 kg of weight
- 20 mL/kg/day for the weight over 20 kg

For example, a child weighing 20 kg has a maintenance fluid requirement of $(100 \times 10) + (50 \times 10) = 1500$ mL. To correct dehydration, the fluid deficit should be calculated using the following formula — volume to be replaced in addition to maintenance = percentage dehydration $\times$ weight (kg) $\times$ 10. This replacement volume should be given over 48 hours. For example, if this 20 kg child has 5% dehydration, he would need 1000 mL $(20 \times 5 \times 10)$ given over 48 hours. This would mean they need 2000 mL per 24 hours (daily maintenance + half of the deficit), which equates to a rate of 83 mL/hour.

Children with clinical dehydration (without shock) should be given oral rehydration solution (ORS). The World Health Organisation recommends ORS at 75 mL/kg every 4 hours. This may be given via a nasogastric tube if the child is unable to drink or if they persistently vomit. Intravenous therapy is required if the child deteriorates despite ORS or if the ORS is not tolerated. Anti-diarrhoeal agents (e.g. loperamide) are not recommended in children.

11. C

Deformities of the head soon after delivery are a common feature in neonates and are rarely a cause for concern. A cephalohaematoma is a haemorrhage that occurs between the periosteum and the skull. As it is bound by the periosteum, it does not cross suture lines. It is more common in patients born by instrumental delivery (forceps or ventouse) and it may increase in size after birth. As the blood gets reabsorbed, it can cause or exacerbate neonatal jaundice.

The most common cause of a skull deformity after birth is due to cranial moulding. This is when the skull bones overlap to reduce the diameter of the skull as it passes through the birth canal. After a few days, the bones should move back into their normal positions and the fontanelles will close as the child grows older. Caput succedaneum is a diffuse collection of sub-cutaneous fluid within the scalp. It has poorly defined margins and may cross suture lines. It tends to resolve over a few days. A subgaleal haemorrhage is a rare but serious condition where a bleed occurs between the aponeurosis of the scalp and the periosteum. It forms a lump that crosses suture lines and it may cause life-threatening blood loss. Craniosynostosis is a condition in which one or more of the sutures close prematurely leading to distorted growth of the skull. This can be resolved surgically.

12. B

The muscular dystrophies are a group of X-linked recessive disorders caused by deletion of the dystrophin gene. A deficiency of dystrophin leads to myocyte necrosis and a consequent release of creatinine kinase. There is progressive muscle degeneration, which presents between 1 and 3 years of age with delayed walking and a waddling gait. Children may be unable to climb stairs without help. Duchenne muscular dystrophy is the most common and most severe subtype. Patients often lose the ability to walk by the age of 12 years. This may be followed by dilated cardiomyopathy and respiratory failure due to weakening of the muscles of respiration. Patients usually die by the age of 20–30 years due to cardiac or respiratory failure. The 'bulky' calves is describing pseudohypertrophy — a phenomenon in which the atrophied muscles have been replaced by fat and fibrous tissue.

Becker muscular dystrophy has similar symptoms to Duchenne muscular dystrophy, but is milder, progresses more slowly, and presents later.

Patients with Becker muscular dystrophy have a normal life expectancy. Myotonic dystrophy is an autosomal dominant trinucleotide repeat disorder that can present at any age but is the most common subtype of muscular dystrophy presenting in adulthood. There are two main types of myotonic dystrophy. Type 1 is more common and more severe and tends to cause muscle weakness and wasting of the legs, hands, neck, and face whereas type 2 tends to affect the shoulders, elbows, and hips. Muscles become myotonic (i.e. unable to relax) wherein patients may also have cataracts, learning disabilities, and arrhythmias. Spinal muscular atrophy is an autosomal recessive condition characterised by degeneration of the anterior horn cells resulting in progressive weakness and wasting of the skeletal muscles. Charcot–Marie–Tooth (CMT) disease is an autosomal dominant peripheral neuropathy in which patients develop symmetrical, slowly progressive distal muscle wasting.

13. D

Viral meningitis is much more common than bacterial meningitis. It is a self-limiting disease with a milder course and less florid symptoms. Viral meningitis is most commonly caused by enteroviruses (e.g. Coxsackie and Echovirus). Viral meningitis is also referred to as aseptic meningitis due to the inability to demonstrate the presence of bacteria. Herpes simplex can cause both meningitis and encephalitis. *Neisseria meningitidis* and *Streptococcus pneumoniae* are the main causes of bacterial meningitis. *Haemophilus influenzae* is a rare cause of bacterial meningitis thanks to the childhood vaccination programme.

14. B

Tetralogy of Fallot (ToF) is a congenital cyanotic heart disease consisting of four anatomical defects: pulmonary stenosis, right ventricular hypertrophy, overriding aorta, and ventricular septal defect (VSD). ToF presents within the first few months of life with hypercyanotic 'tet' spells in which the child has episodes of central cyanosis while crying or feeding. Examination may reveal an ejection systolic murmur due to pulmonary stenosis. A chest X-ray may show a characteristic small heart with an up-tilted apex and pulmonary artery bay, creating a 'boot-shaped' heart with decreased pulmonary vascular markings. Prolonged hypercyanotic spells can be treated with propranolol, morphine, and fluids. Definitive surgical treatment is usually performed at 6 months to close the VSD and relieve the right ventricular outflow obstruction.

Transposition of the great arteries is another type of congenital cyanotic heart disease characterised by reversal of the aorta and pulmonary artery, meaning that oxygenated blood returns to the lungs rather than the body. This is incompatible with life and presents with severe cyanosis within the first few days of life as the ductus arteriosus closes. Persistent ductus arteriosus (PDA), atrial septal defect (ASD), and VSD are examples of acyanotic congenital heart disease. VSD is the most common and may present with signs of heart failure and a pansytolic murmur at the lower left sternal edge. PDA causes a subclavicular continuous murmur, bounding pulse, left subclavicular thrill, widened pulse pressure, and signs of heart failure. ASD can cause an ejection systolic murmur at the upper left sternal edge and a fixed and widely-split second heart sound.

15. A

Marfan syndrome is an autosomal dominant disorder of the connective tissue. Patients tend to be tall and slender with disproportionately long limbs. They also tend to have a long, narrow face with a high-arched palate. Other features include joint hypermobility, scoliosis, flat feet, and pectus excavatum. Patients are at increased risk of cardiac abnormalities (e.g. mitral prolapse, aortic aneurysms, and aortic dissection) and visual disturbances (e.g. cataracts, lens dislocation).

As a general rule, autosomal dominant disorders tend to affect structural proteins, whereas autosomal recessive disorders tend to affect metabolic pathways. Meiotic non-disjunction describes failure of chromosomes to separate properly during cell division and is responsible for trisomies (e.g. Down syndrome) and sex chromosome aneuploidies (e.g. Turner syndrome). The table shows some of the most common inherited disorders and their inheritance pattern.

Autosome recessive	Autosomal dominant
Cystic fibrosis	Ehlers Danlos syndrome
Homocystinuria	Myotonic dystrophy
Sickle cell disease	Neurofibromatosis
Thalassaemia	Noonan syndrome
Phenylketonuria	Osteogenesis imperfecta
Spinal muscular atrophy	Tuberous sclerosis
Friedreich ataxia (an exception to the 'metabolic' rule for autosomal recessive disorders)	Achondroplasia
X-linked recessive	**X-linked dominant**
Duchenne and Becker muscular dystrophy	Fragile X syndrome
Haemophilia A and B	Rett syndrome
Glucose-6-phosphate dehydrogenase deficiency	

16. C

Acute otitis media (AOM) is inflammation of the middle ear usually due to infection. Older children will complain of earache and younger children will hold, tug, or rub their ear and have non-specific features such as fever, crying, poor feeding, and irritability. Otoscopy will demonstrate a red, yellow, or cloudy tympanic membrane that may be bulging or perforated. There may be discharge in the external auditory canal and an air-fluid level behind the tympanic membrane, indicating a middle ear effusion. AOM can be caused by both viruses (e.g. RSV, rhinovirus, adenovirus) and bacteria (e.g. *Haemophilus influenzae, Streptococcus pneumoniae*). Parents can be reassured and advised that it usually resolves spontaneously within 3–7 days and that paracetamol or ibuprofen can be given if the child is irritable. Antibiotics may be considered in cases of bilateral AOM in children under the age of 2 years, if symptoms do not resolve within 3 days, or if there are co-existing conditions (e.g. cystic fibrosis). The antibiotic regimen of choice is a 5–7 day course of amoxicillin. If symptoms worsen, children should be assessed for complications (e.g. glue ear, hearing loss, perforation, mastoiditis). An ENT referral is necessary in children who have failed to respond to two courses of antibiotics, those with suspected glue ear and in recurrent AOM that is unexplained, associated with complications or a craniofacial abnormality (e.g. Down syndrome).

17. B

Developmental dysplasia of the hip (DDH) is normally picked up during neonatal screening, however, if missed, it may present several years later with an abnormal gait (waddling or toe walking), limited hip abduction, leg length discrepancy, and asymmetrical skin folds on the affected side. The newborn examination, performed within 72 hours of birth, screens for DDH using two manoeuvres. Firstly, the Barlow manoeuvre which determines whether the hip can be dislocated posteriorly, followed by the Ortolani manoeuvre which determines whether the hip can be replaced into the acetabulum. These are repeated at 6–8 weeks and an ultrasound scan is the preferred investigation in babies aged 6 weeks to 6 months to confirm clinical findings. An ultrasound may be recommended in the presence of a normal examination if risk factors are present, such as a family history of DDH, breech presentation, multiple pregnancy, and prematurity. Foreign countries may have a different neonatal screening programme so patients born abroad may present late. Beyond 6 months of age, hip radiographs are preferred over ultrasound and are warranted if the hip examination is abnormal.

In children under the age of 6 months, DDH can be managed with a Pavlik harness in which the hips are held flexed and abducted for several weeks. Children between 18 months and 6 years are treated surgically via open reduction in which any obstructing tissues are removed to allow the femoral head to be relocated into the acetabulum. Children over the age of 6 years are less amenable to open reduction and reconstruction so may require a salvage osteotomy.

18. B

Respiratory distress syndrome (RDS) is caused by insufficient surfactant production and is more common in preterm infants. It presents within the first few hours of life with signs of respiratory distress, such as tachypnoea, expiratory grunting, nasal flaring, cyanosis, and chest recession. Risk factors for RDS include male sex, caesarean section, maternal diabetes mellitus, and multiple pregnancy and are associated with other abnormalities, such as necrotising enterocolitis, patent ductus arteriosus, and hypoglycaemia. Chest X-ray will typically show bilateral and symmetrical ground-glass shadowing and air bronchograms. Antenatal glucocorticoids are given if preterm delivery is anticipated to stimulate foetal surfactant production and prevent RDS. Otherwise it is treated with exogenous surfactant and oxygen therapy.

Transient tachypnoea of the newborn is the most common cause of respiratory distress in term infants and occurs due to a delay in the resorption of amniotic fluid in the lungs. It most commonly occurs following caesarean section and settles within the first day of life. Meconium aspiration can result in mechanical obstruction and a chemical pneumonitis, resulting in areas of collapse and consolidation on chest X-ray. It is more common in post-term newborns. Bronchopulmonary dysplasia describes pathological lung changes in infants following prolonged artificial ventilation.

19. B

Constipation is very common in young children and tends to be accompanied by faecal impaction. Patients may also present with soiling or overflow diarrhoea. It is important to assess psychological factors that could be contributing to constipation, as anxiety about clean toilets is a common factor leading to constipation in children. Constipation leads to a vicious cycle of a stool being hard and difficult to pass, resulting in painful passage which reinforces faecal retention. When assessing a constipated child, it is important to feel for a faecal mass as its presence would indicate the need for a disimpaction regimen of osmotic laxatives. The 1st line treatment for constipation in children is polyethylene glycol and electrolytes (also known as Movicol). This may be given as a disimpaction regime (escalating dose over 2 weeks) or a maintenance dose (same dose every day). The laxatives should continue to be used until normal bowel habit is re-established. If this is ineffective, a stimulant laxative (e.g.

Senna) should be added. Behavioural approaches (e.g. positive reward system) can also be advised to facilitate toileting.

20. A

Cerebral palsy is a permanent disorder of movement, posture, and motor function due to a non-progressive lesion of the developing brain. There are four types of cerebral palsy, of which spastic cerebral palsy makes up 70–80% of cases. Spastic cerebral palsy is caused by a lesion in the motor cortex and is characterised by spasticity and hypertonia. It is further sub-divided into hemiplegic (involving one arm and leg on the same side with facial sparing), quadriplegic (involving all four limbs with truncal hypotonia) and diplegic (involving all four limbs, but the legs are affected more than the arms). This patient has left-sided hypertonia with a normal right side, suggesting that this is spastic hemiplegic cerebral palsy.

Dyskinetic cerebral palsy is caused by a lesion in the basal ganglia. It is characterised by variable muscle tone and movements that are involuntary and stereotyped such as chorea, athetosis, and dystonia. Ataxic cerebral palsy is caused by a cerebellar lesion and is characterised by a lack of voluntary coordination of muscle movements presenting as intention tremor, ataxic gait, and speech abnormalities. Mixed cerebral palsy is caused by lesions in more than one location, resulting in children presenting with features of more than one type of cerebral palsy.

21. C

Erythema multiforme is a rash caused by a hypersensitivity reaction, usually to viral infections such as herpes simplex virus. Other causes of erythema multiforme include bacteria (e.g. *Mycoplasma*) and medications (e.g. sulphonamide antibiotics). The management of erythema multiforme depends on the aetiology — if present, triggers should be removed, otherwise the disease is typically self-limiting and will resolve over time.

Guttate psoriasis also often follows a streptococcal throat infection or an upper respiratory tract viral infection, but presents with small, raindrop-like, scaly patches on the trunk and upper limbs. Pityriasis versicolor is a yeast infection of the skin caused by *Malassezia furfur*. It causes pale patches in those with pigmented skin and pink patches in unpigmented skin. Tinea (also known as ringworm) is a fungal skin infection that is named based on the body part affected — tinea pedis (foot infection), tinea corporis (body infection), and tinea cruris (groin infection). Tinea causes characteristic annular (round) scaly patches that are often less red and scaly in the centre. Miliaria (sweat rash) is caused by obstruction of the sweat ducts and is common in neonates. It presents with small clear blisters that are widely spread on the head, neck, and trunk.

22. B

This infant has bronchiolitis — an infection of the epithelial lining of the lower bronchial tree, most commonly caused by respiratory syncytial virus (RSV). Bronchiolitis affects children aged under 2 years, with a peak incidence between 3 and 6 months. It presents with a coryzal prodrome lasting 1–3 days followed by a persistent dry cough and a high-pitched expiratory wheeze. Other symptoms include poor feeding and fever. Examination findings include tachypnoea, chest recession, and fine inspiratory crackles.

Any children with bronchiolitis who have any of the following features should be admitted to hospital: apnoea, oxygen saturation less than 92% on air, less than 50% of usual fluid intake, and persistent severe respiratory distress. Please note that assessing fluid intake as a percentage of usual may be misleading as many babies are overfed. Oxygen should be given to children if their oxygen saturation is consistently less than 92% on air and intravenous fluids should only be given to children who cannot tolerate oral feeds or have impending respiratory failure. Upper airway suctioning should be considered in children who have respiratory distress or feeding difficulties because of upper airway secretions. The infant in this case does not require any of these interventions, so is safe to be discharged once he is clinically stable, is taking adequate oral fluids, and has maintained oxygen saturation over 92% on air. The parents should be advised to use paracetamol or ibuprofen if the child is irritable and to monitor regularly for the aforementioned red flag symptoms. Palivizumab is a monoclonal antibody that is used to prevent RSV infection in children who are at risk of severe disease.

23. B

Haemolytic uraemic syndrome (HUS) is a condition characterised by a triad of microangiopathic haemolytic anaemia (e.g. pallor), thrombocytopenia (e.g. bruising), and acute renal failure (e.g. reduced urine output). This is a thrombotic microangiopathy that follows infection with shiga toxin-producing *Escherichia coli* O157 and *Shigella dysenteriae*. Patients typically have a prodrome of bloody diarrhoea, fever, abdominal cramps, and vomiting followed by the features of HUS which develop 5–10 days later. Thrombotic thrombocytopenic purpura (TTP) is another thrombotic microangiopathy which results in failure to break down large multimers of von Willebrand factor, leading to fibrin deposition in small vessels. TTP has the same features of HUS along with fever and neurological symptoms.

Henoch–Schönlein purpura is an IgA vasculitis which presents with a triad of purpuric rash over the extensor surfaces, arthralgia, and abdominal pain. Complications include glomerulonephritis leading to nephritic syndrome (proteinuria, haematuria, oliguria, and hypertension). IgA nephropathy and post-streptococcal glomerulonephritis can also cause nephritic syndrome — IgA nephropathy presents 1–2 days following an upper respiratory tract infection, whereas post-streptococcal glomerulonephritis presents 1–3 weeks following a streptococcal throat infection.

24. C

Delayed puberty is the absence of pubertal development by the age of 14 years in girls and 15 years in boys. Causes can be divided into hypogonadotrophic hypogonadism (low FSH and LH) and hypergonadotrophic hypogonadism (high FSH and LH). Delayed puberty is much more common in boys and is typically hypogonadotrophic due to constitutional delay. A family history of delayed puberty is often present. Some other causes of hypogonadotrophic hypogonadism include systemic diseases (e.g. cystic fibrosis) and hypothalamic-pituitary disorders (e.g. isolated gonadotrophin deficiency). Hypergonadotrophic hypogonadism is caused by gonadal damage or dysfunction which may be due to chemotherapy, irradiation, trauma, surgery, chromosomal abnormalities (e.g. Klinefelter syndrome), and androgen insensitivity syndrome. Klinefelter syndrome is a condition in which males have two or more X chromosomes. This manifests with gynaecomastia, a feminised physique, small testes, and a tall stature. Klinefelter syndrome leads to hypogonadism, resulting in a low testosterone and elevated gonadotrophins.

Androgen insensitivity syndrome is caused by end-organ resistance to testosterone in which genotypically male children have a female phenotype. These children may present with primary amenorrhoea, delayed puberty, and groin swellings (undescended testes). Kallmann syndrome is characterised by anosmia and a failure of gonadotrophin-releasing hormone production resulting in low testosterone and low gonadotrophins. Low gonadotrophins and elevated testosterone suggest that there is a gonadotrophin-independent source of testosterone (e.g. adrenal or testicular tumour) causing precocious puberty. Elevated TSH and low T4 is suggestive of hypothyroidism, which may affect the onset of puberty and cause symptoms such as weight gain, constipation, and cold insensitivity.

25. B

The nasal influenza vaccine is offered annually to all primary school children in the UK. Children with long-term health conditions such as diabetes mellitus and asthma are at increased risk of developing serious complications of influenza, so they should be offered the vaccine up to adulthood. It is important to note whether a child has an egg allergy before administering the vaccine, as the IM and nasal influenza vaccines both contain egg-based components. It is recommended that children who have only a mild reaction to egg (e.g. hives) should receive the vaccine in a primary care setting. If they have a more serious reaction to egg (e.g. anaphylaxis), a discussion should be had about the risks and benefits of giving the vaccine, and if it is decided to administer the vaccine, it should be done in hospital under specialist supervision with the tools to treat an anaphylactic reaction. As the child in this question has asthma, they should be considered for the IM influenza vaccine. Furthermore, as his egg allergy only causes hives, it would be safe to administer the vaccine in a primary care setting.

26. A

Toddler's diarrhoea is the most common cause of persistent loose stools in children. Patients will have frequent loose stools which often contain small amounts of undigested foods, such as carrots, sweetcorn, and peas. Children are otherwise well and growing normally. The condition usually resolves by the age of 5 years and it is managed with dietary interventions, such as reducing intake of refined sugars and avoiding excessive fluid and fibre intake.

Cows' milk protein allergy usually develops when cows' milk is first introduced into the diet or through the transfer of cows' milk protein allergens in breastmilk. It presents with a wide range of symptoms, such as rashes, diarrhoea, vomiting, and hay fever-like symptoms. Infantile colic is defined as inconsolable crying or screaming, often accompanied by drawing up of the knees and passage of excessive flatus that occurs for more than 3 hours per day for more than 3 days per week for more than 3 weeks. It is a benign condition with no identifiable organic cause. Diarrhoea is the most common symptom of coeliac disease, along with abdominal pain, bloating, flatulence, and constipation. Coeliac disease is an important differential to consider in children with diarrhoea, particularly those with growth faltering and anaemia. Rotavirus is the most common cause of infantile gastroenteritis and usually presents with fever and vomiting, followed by diarrhoea that lasts for 3–8 days. Its prevalence has decreased significantly since the introduction of the rotavirus vaccine.

27. C

Cyanosis within the first few days of life is highly suggestive of congenital cyanotic heart disease. There are three main diseases that are classified as congenital cyanotic heart disease: transposition of the great arteries (TGA), tetralogy of Fallot (TOF), and tricuspid atresia. This patient most likely has TGA given the early onset of cyanosis and the inability to achieve sufficient oxygen saturations despite being given a high concentration of oxygen. TGA is a rare condition in which the aorta and pulmonary arteries are reversed. This, in effect, means that there are two independent circulations — one from the left side of the heart to the lungs, and another from the right side of the heart to the rest of the body. Infants are able to survive initially due to a patent ductus arteriosus allowing the blood from these two circulations to mix. However, as the ductus arteriosus closes in the days after birth, the blood is no longer able to mix leading to profound cyanosis and low oxygen saturations. The immediate management involves starting a prostaglandin infusion (e.g. alprostadil) to maintain the patency of the ductus arteriosus. This buys time before definitive surgical correction can be arranged. The main side-effect of prostaglandin infusions is apnoea, so many neonates will require intubation. A chest X-ray would reveal an 'egg on a string' appearance and a hyperoxia test will reveal failure to increase partial pressure of oxygen despite receiving a high concentration of oxygen.

28. D

Fragile X syndrome is an X-linked dominant condition caused by a trinucleotide repeat. It affects both males and females, but has a much milder phenotype in females. Most children with fragile X syndrome have a learning disability, anxiety, ADHD, or autism. Characteristic physical features include a long, narrow face, large ears with a prominent jaw and forehead, high-arched palate, flat feet, and macro-orchidism. Children are at risk of mitral valve prolapse (causing a pansystolic murmur), epilepsy, strabismus, and infertility. Some of the characteristics of other eponymous syndromes are as follows.

Syndrome	Features
DiGeorge syndrome	Cleft palate, learning disabilities, thymic aplasia, developmental delay, hypocalcaemia, cardiac abnormalities (interrupted aortic arch, tetralogy of Fallot)
Down syndrome	Flat nasal bridge, upslanted palpebral fissures, Brushfield spots, low set ears, epicanthal folds, short stature, single palmar crease, hypotonia, congenital heart defects (AVSD), duodenal atresia, Hirschsprung disease, leukaemia, atlantoaxial instability
Noonan syndrome	Coarse facial features, webbed neck, short stature, pectus excavatum, learning disabilities, pulmonary valve stenosis

(Continued)

(*Continued*)

Syndrome	Features
Patau syndrome	Microcephaly, cleft palate, dysplastic ears, polydactyly, undescended testes, cardiac, renal, and visual abnormalities
Pierre Robin sequence	Triad of micrognathia, cleft palate, and glossoptosis
Prader–Willi syndrome	Hypotonia, almond-shaped eyes, behavioural problems, hypogonadism, hyperphagia, obesity
Williams syndrome	Elfin facies, learning disabilities, supravalvular aortic stenosis, friendly and extroverted personality, neonatal hypercalcaemia

29. D

A neuroblastoma is a tumour that arises from primitive neural crest cells and can occur anywhere along the sympathetic chain, but most frequently develops in the adrenal glands. The majority of cases occur in children under 10 years of age. They typically present with a large abdominal mass and may have signs of metastatic disease. Spinal cord metastases can lead to weakness and numbness, and orbital metastases can cause eye changes. Other features of metastatic disease include hepatomegaly, cutaneous lesions, and skeletal pain. Since this is a malignancy of the adrenal medulla, most patients will have elevated levels of urinary catecholamine by-products, such as homovanillic acid (HVA) and vanillylmandelic acid (VMA). A biopsy is required for a definitive diagnosis and a MIBG scan is used to look for metastases.

The red reflex is a component of the newborn examination and refers to the normal red colour that is reflected from the back of a healthy eye when observed with an ophthalmoscope. An absent or reduced red reflex may indicate the presence of a congenital cataract, corneal or retinal scarring, haemorrhage or retinoblastoma. Reed–Sternberg cells are bi-nucleate giant cells with prominent nucleoli (resembling an 'owl's eye' appearance) and are seen in core or excisional biopsies from patients with Hodgkin's lymphoma. Acute lymphoblastic leukaemia is characterised by the presence of more than 20% lymphoblasts in the bone marrow. These lymphoblasts may spill into the peripheral circulation. 'Onion skinning' is a periosteal reaction characterised by the formation of concentric layers of new bone and is suggestive of Ewing sarcoma — the second most common malignant primary bone tumour of childhood (after osteosarcoma).

30. A

Non-accidental injury (NAI) can have a variety of presentations, listed in the following table.

Type of abuse	Manifestations
Physical	Bruising, fractures, torn frenulum, drowsiness (subdural haematoma)
Sexual	Anal/genital soreness, recurrent UTI, discharge
Neglect	Unkempt, failure to interact appropriately with healthcare services (e.g. missed vaccines)

The median age of a baby being able to roll over is 4 months, which means that it is highly unlikely that the 2-month-old boy in this SBA had, in fact, rolled off the changing table. Furthermore, the presence of two bruises on one arm does not seem to fit the type of injury that is likely to have been incurred after falling from a table. Whenever there is any doubt regarding the circumstances of an injury, the child should be admitted, and senior colleagues should be informed. It is also essential to inform the child safeguarding team at the hospital, who may involve social services and the police if necessary.

Paediatrics: Paper 2

Questions

1. A 2-day-old neonate on the postnatal ward has been feeding poorly and has a temperature of 37.3°C. A septic screen is requested. Which empirical antibiotic treatment would be most appropriate to commence in this situation?

   A Amoxicillin
   B Ceftriaxone and vancomycin
   C Benzylpenicillin and gentamicin
   D Co-amoxiclav
   E Doxycycline

2. A 3-year-old boy has had a severe bout of diarrhoea and vomiting. Several other children at his nursery have also had similar symptoms. Which of the following causes of gastroenteritis should be reported to the Health Protection Unit?

   A Rotavirus
   B *Campylobacter jejuni*
   C Norovirus
   D *Staphylococcus aureus*
   E *Clostridium difficile*

3. A 12-year-old boy has had a 10-week history of joint pain. On examination, his proximal interphalangeal joints, wrists, and knees are tender, swollen, and stiff. He has also experienced some difficulty swallowing and has a temperature of 38.2°C. What is the most likely diagnosis?

    A Reactive arthritis
    B Oligoarticular juvenile idiopathic arthritis
    C Polyarticular juvenile idiopathic arthritis
    D Systemic arthritis
    E Septic arthritis

4. A 4-month-old boy is brought to see his GP with concerns about a persistent nappy rash. His mother explains that the rash has persisted despite switching to high absorbency nappies, changing nappies frequently and cleaning the skin with alcohol-free baby wipes. On examination, the rash is well demarcated, erythematous and is sparing the skin folds. The child has become increasingly irritable over as the rash has progressed. What is the most appropriate management for this child?

    A Continue with self-management strategies and review in 2 weeks
    B Advise on barrier protection
    C Advise on barrier protection and prescribe topical hydrocortisone 1%
    D Advise against barrier protection and prescribe a topical imidazole cream
    E Prescribe oral flucloxacillin

5. A 16-year-old girl with a past medical history of infantile spasms, autism, and learning difficulties, has developed depigmented patches on her skin with angiofibromata in a butterfly distribution across the bridge of her nose. A CT scan identifies polycystic kidneys and cardiac rhabdomyomas. What is the most likely underlying diagnosis?

A Sturge–Weber syndrome
B Tuberous sclerosis
C Rett syndrome
D Neurofibromatosis type 1
E Neurofibromatosis type 2

6. Which of the following regarding sudden infant death syndrome is true?

   A The peak age range is 1–2 years
   B Low birthweight is a risk factor
   C It is more common in girls
   D It is safe to sleep in the same bed as the infant
   E It usually occurs while the infant is awake

7. A 9-month-old boy has vomited three times in the last 24 hours and has seemed more irritable over the past few days. His mother has also had to change his nappy more frequently than usual. A urine dipstick is positive for nitrites and leukocytes, so a urinary tract infection is diagnosed. He developed a similar episode, diagnosed as pyelonephritis, 2 months ago. How should this child be investigated?

   A DMSA within 4–6 months of acute infection
   B Ultrasound scan during the acute infection
   C Ultrasound scan within 6 weeks of acute infection
   D Ultrasound scan during the acute infection and DMSA within 6 weeks
   E Ultrasound scan within 6 weeks of acute infection and DMSA within 4–6 months

8. A 2-year-old boy is brought to A&E with a 24-hour history of a barking cough and snotty nose. On examination, a quiet stridor is heard with mild sternal recession. What is the most appropriate management option for this patient?

    A Inhaled beclomethasone
    B Inhaled salbutamol
    C Oral prednisolone
    D Oral dexamethasone
    E Nebulised adrenaline

9. A 7-year-old boy has developed some pubic hair and acne. On examination, his penis is enlarged, and both testes have a volume of 7 mL
(<4 mL). There is sparse hair growth at the base of the penis. He is
on the 51st centile for height and weight. What is the most likely
diagnosis?

    A McCune Albright syndrome
    B Congenital adrenal hyperplasia
    C Leydig cell testicular tumour
    D Adrenal tumour
    E Hypothalamic hamartomas

10. A 15-year-old girl presents to A&E with sudden-onset abdominal
pain and vomiting. On examination, she appears unwell and has a
fever of 39.5°C. There is generalised tenderness and bowel sounds
are absent. She had experienced some milder lower abdominal
discomfort and nausea the previous day. What is the most likely
diagnosis?

    A Appendicular mass
    B Appendicular abscess
    C Bowel obstruction
    D Perforated appendix
    E Ectopic pregnancy

11. A 5-year-old boy is brought to see his GP after developing a rash on
his buttocks. On inspection, there are several scaly, annular lesions
across both buttocks. The child is otherwise well but has been complaining about the rash being itchy. Given the most likely diagnosis,
what is the most appropriate treatment option?

    A Topical terbinafine
    B Topical ketoconazole
    C Topical clobetasol propionate
    D Oral itraconazole
    E Oral prednisolone

12. A 2-week-old newborn with Down syndrome has developed shortness of breath. He has also been struggling to feed during this period and has not been gaining weight. On examination, he is tachypnoeic, tachycardic and his liver is 4 cm below the costal margin. No murmur is heard on auscultation of the precordium. What is the most likely diagnosis?

    A Ventricular septal defect
    B Atrioventricular septal defect
    C Atrial septal defect
    D Tricuspid atresia
    E Interrupted aortic arch

13. A 4-year-old girl presents to her GP with a sore throat and a temperature of 38.2°C. On examination, there are blisters on the dorsal and palmar surfaces of the hands and feet, and small ulcers in the mouth and on the palate. What is the most likely diagnosis?

    A Molluscum contagiosum
    B Herpangina
    C Roseola infantum
    D Quinsy
    E Hand, foot and mouth disease

14. A 4-year-old boy with sickle cell disease presents to A&E with painful swelling of the hands. On examination, there is restricted range of motion and the fingers are oedematous, tender, and warm. His vital signs are shown below:

Heart rate: 136 bpm
Respiratory rate: 24 breaths/min

Temperature: 38.5°C
Blood pressure: 100/68 mmHg
Oxygen saturation: 98% on air

How should this child be managed?

A Advise on pain relief and discharge
B Advise on pain relief and give penicillin V and discharge
C Give analgesia and admit
D Give analgesia and hydroxycarbamide and admit
E Give analgesia and corticosteroids and admit

15. A 5-year-old girl presents to the GP with bloating and diarrhoea. Her mum explains that a few weeks ago she was unwell with a fever, diarrhoea, and vomiting that lasted 3 days. These symptoms initially resolved, but the diarrhoea started again, and she complained of feeling bloated when her normal diet was reintroduced. What is the most likely diagnosis?

A Irritable bowel syndrome
B Giardiasis
C Inflammatory bowel disease
D Mesenteric adenitis
E Shigellosis

16. A 7-year-old boy continues to wet the bed about 3 times per week. He has no daytime symptoms and has never been dry at night. No abnormalities are detected on the urine dipstick. What is the most appropriate 1st line management option?

A Advise regarding fluid intake and suggest a reward system only
B Advise regarding fluid intake, suggest a reward system and offer an enuresis alarm
C Advise regarding fluid intake, suggest a reward system and offer desmopressin
D Advise regarding fluid intake, offer desmopressin and an enuresis alarm
E Refer to secondary care or an enuresis clinic

17. A 4-year-old boy is brought into A&E after he rapidly developed several small painful blisters on his face. The blisters are widespread, monomorphic and filled with a yellow liquid. The child has also developed a fever and complains of feeling unwell. He has a history of eczema for which he frequently applies emollients. What is the most likely diagnosis?

    A *Staphylococcus aureus* infection
    B *Streptococcus pyogenes* infection
    C Varicella zoster infection
    D Herpes simplex infection
    E Parvovirus B19 infection

18. A 4-year-old girl presents to the GP with her mum who is concerned because her vagina looks abnormal. She is otherwise well and has no issues with urination. On examination, there is partial labial fusion. How should this child be managed?

    A Arrange surgical separation
    B Prescribe topical oestrogen
    C Reassure and arrange follow-up
    D Advise regular manual separation
    E Prescribe topical hydrocortisone

19. A 2-week-old boy is admitted to hospital as he has been vomiting regularly since birth. He has also lost more weight than expected at this stage. On examination, his fontanelle is depressed, his skin turgor is poor, and his penis appears enlarged. A hormone profile reveals an elevated 17α-hydroxyprogesterone level. Which biochemical abnormalities would you expect to see in this patient?

    A Metabolic alkalosis, hypoglycaemia, hypokalaemia, and hyponatraemia
    B Metabolic alkalosis, hypoglycaemia, hyperkalaemia, and hyponatraemia
    C Metabolic acidosis, hyperglycaemia, hyperkalaemia, and hyponatraemia

    D Metabolic acidosis, hypoglycaemia, hyperkalaemia, and hyponatraemia

    E Metabolic acidosis, hypoglycaemia, hypokalaemia, and hyponatraemia

20. A 16-year-old girl presents to the GP with a swollen, painful right knee and ankle. She also describes a burning sensation when passing urine, pain in her heels whilst walking and redness and irritation of her eyes. She recently completed a course of antibiotics for a chlamydia infection. What is the most likely diagnosis?

    A Systemic lupus erythematosus
    B Juvenile idiopathic arthritis
    C Kawasaki disease
    D Juvenile dermatomyositis
    E Reactive arthritis

21. A 3-year-old boy is being discharged from hospital after presenting with a febrile convulsion for the third time. What advice should be given to the parents regarding recurrent seizures?

    A Give paracetamol at the onset of the fever to prevent febrile convulsions
    B Give paracetamol at the onset of the seizure
    C Give buccal midazolam at the onset of the seizure and call for an ambulance immediately
    D Give buccal midazolam after 5 minutes if the seizure hasn't stopped and call an ambulance if the seizure has not stopped after a further 5 minutes
    E Give buccal midazolam after 5 minutes and call for an ambulance if the seizure does not terminate immediately

22. A newborn baby girl has had difficulty breathing since her birth 1 hour ago. On examination, there is marked chest recession, the heart sounds are displaced to the right side of the chest with absent air entry on the left. Despite oxygen therapy, her oxygen saturation remains at 81%. What is the most likely diagnosis?

    A Pneumothorax
    B Congenital diaphragmatic hernia
    C Pneumonia
    D Hypoxic ischaemic encephalopathy
    E Oesophageal atresia with tracheal fistula

23. A 2-year-old girl is brought to A&E after becoming drowsy over the past 24 hours. On examination, her respiratory rate is increased, and her breaths are shallow, so a chest X-ray is requested (report below). She has no significant past medical history; however, it is noted that she has not received any vaccinations.

    Temperature: 37.1°C
    Heart rate: 102 bpm
    Respiratory rate: 24 breaths/min
    Blood pressure: 92/62 mm Hg
    CXR: lung fields are clear bilaterally, two right-sided posterior rib fractures

    What is the most appropriate investigation to request next?

        A Blood cultures
        B CT head scan
        C Sputum microscopy
        D Urine microscopy
        E Measles immunoglobulin

24. A 2-year-old boy presents to A&E with his parents after his skin turned yellow and his urine became dark. His mother explains that he has had a fever since yesterday and has been complaining of some tummy pain and stinging when he passes urine. He had neonatal jaundice soon after he was born. The results of his urine dipstick, blood tests, and blood film are shown in the following:

    Urine dipstick: nitrites ++, leukocytes +, blood + and bilirubin ++
    White cell count: 18×10^9/L (5–12)
    Haemoglobin: 104 g/L (110–140)
    Mean cell volume: 85 fL (80–96)

Reticulocytes: 5% (0.5–1.5)
Bilirubin: 25 umol/L (3–17)
Lactate dehydrogenase: 1020 IU/L (400–900)
Blood film: anisocytosis, bite cells, and Heinz bodies

What is the most likely underlying diagnosis?

    A Parvovirus B19 infection
    B Diamond-Blackfan anaemia
    C Hereditary spherocytosis
    D Pyruvate kinase deficiency
    E Glucose-6-phosphate dehydrogenase deficiency

25. A mother of a 12-week-old baby boy presents to her GP with concerns about her baby's feeding. He is exclusively breastfed and vomits after most feeds. The vomitus consists of milk only, appears effortless and the child does not appear significantly distressed. The child was initially growing along the 38th centile but has recently dropped to the 31st centile. A midwife has carried out a breastfeeding assessment and is happy with the mother's technique and the child's latch. What is the most appropriate next step in the management of this patient?

    A Alginate therapy
    B Switch to formula feeds
    C Trial of omeprazole
    D Trial of ranitidine
    E Admit for enteral tube (NGT) feeding

26. A 2-year-old girl has been referred to paediatrics by her GP after a heart murmur was noted on examination. Her parents are advised that it is most likely an innocent murmur. Which of the following is a feature of an innocent murmur?

    A Mild symptoms only
    B Systolic murmurs
    C Radiates to the neck
    D No positional variation
    E Loudest at the apex

27. A 3-year-old girl is able to walk independently but cannot hop on one leg, draws random marks with a crayon but cannot copy a line or circle, says 'mama' and 'dada' but no other words, and can feed herself with a spoon. Which developmental domain is delayed?

   A Gross motor
   B Vision and fine motor
   C Hearing, speech and language
   D Social, emotional and behavioural
   E Normal variant

28. A 7-year-old girl has developed a widespread maculopapular rash. She has been complaining of pain when swallowing and has had a fever for the past 3 days. On examination, the rash is widespread with an abrasive texture, there are enlarged papilla on the tongue and cervical lymphadenopathy. Her vital signs are shown below:

   Heart rate: 106 bpm
   Respiratory rate: 22 breaths/min
   Temperature: 38.2°C
   Blood pressure: 108/70 mm Hg

   What is the most appropriate management option?

   A Reassure and discharge with advice regarding pain relief
   B Admit to hospital for antibiotic therapy
   C Admit to hospital to receive high-dose aspirin and IVIG
   D Prescribe phenoxymethylpenicillin and recommend school exclusion for 24 hours after starting antibiotics
   E Prescribe azithromycin and recommend school exclusion for 48 hours after starting antibiotics

29. A 5-year-old boy who has recently moved to the UK is brought to see his GP after his mother noticed a lump sticking out of his rectum when he goes to the toilet. The lump doesn't appear to cause him any distress and can be manually reduced. He has a past medical history of recurrent chest infections, the most recent of which was treated by antibiotics in hospital 3 weeks ago. On examination, he is small for

his age and shows some degree of conjunctival pallor. What is the most likely diagnosis?

A Hirschsprung disease
B Connective tissue disorder
C Primary ciliary dyskinesia
D Cystic fibrosis
E Chronic constipation

30. A 4-year-old boy is rushed into A&E with an itchy rash and breathing difficulties. It started soon after eating a slice of cake at a birthday party. Suspecting an anaphylactic reaction, two doses of IM adrenaline have been administered by the paramedics and the breathing difficulties have settled. On examination, there is widespread urticaria, angioedema of the lips, and a widespread wheeze. His observations are shown in the following:

Heart rate: 162 bpm
Respiratory rate: 36 breaths/min
Temperature: 37.4°C
Blood pressure: 62/44 mm Hg
Oxygen saturation: 89% on air

How else should this child be managed?

A Administer oxygen, give a rapid fluid challenge, give IV chlorphenamine, and IV hydrocortisone
B Administer oxygen, give a rapid fluid challenge, give IV chlorphenamine, and oral prednisolone
C Administer oxygen and nebulised salbutamol, give a rapid fluid challenge, give IV chlorphenamine, and IV hydrocortisone
D Administer oxygen and nebulised salbutamol, give a rapid fluid challenge, give IV chlorphenamine, and oral prednisolone
E Administer oxygen and nebulised adrenaline, give a rapid fluid challenge, give IV chlorphenamine, and oral prednisolone

Answers

1. C

This neonate has developed early-onset sepsis. The exact definition of early-onset sepsis varies — some sources will define it as sepsis developing within the first 72 hours, whereas others will include sepsis up to 7 days of life. Features of sepsis in a neonate can be variable and relatively non-specific such as reduced activity, poor feeding, and jaundice. A fever may not be present in neonates as their immune system may be too immature to mount a fever. Neonates may, however, have temperature instability in which their temperature fluctuates, and they may become hypothermic. At this age, there is a very low threshold for treating neonates with IV antibiotics and the presence of risk factors (e.g. prematurity, maternal, prelabour rupture of membranes) may lower the threshold further. Early-onset sepsis is caused by bacteria that are transmitted to the neonate during their passage through the birth canal. The most commonly implicated organisms are Group B *Streptococcus*, *Escherichia coli*, and *Listeria monocytogenes*. The antibiotics used to treat early-onset sepsis may vary depending on the trust, but they typically include a penicillin (e.g. benzylpenicillin) and an aminoglycoside (e.g. gentamicin) to cover Gram-negatives.

2. B

There are many notifiable diseases that affect children. The following diarrhoeal diseases should be reported to the Health Protection Unit: *Campylobacter jejuni*, *Listeria monocytogenes*, *Escherichia coli* O157, *Shigella* and *Salmonella*.

3. C

Juvenile idiopathic arthritis (JIA) refers to persistent joint swelling lasting longer than 6 weeks in patients under the age of 16 years. There are seven subtypes of JIA of which the four main subtypes are outlined in the following table.

The other three subtypes of JIA are psoriatic JIA (arthritis and psoriasis), enthesitis-related JIA, and undifferentiated JIA. This patient is presenting

Subtype	Epidemiology	Pattern of joint involvement	Extra-articular features	Laboratory findings
Oligoarticular JIA	Most common subtype Peak incidence is 2–4 years	Maximum of four joints. Asymmetrical, affecting large joints (e.g. knees, ankles)	Chronic anterior uveitis, leg length discrepancy	ANA positive RF negative ESR elevated
Seronegative polyarticular JIA	30% of cases Bimodal incidence (1–4 years and 6–12 years)	Involving 5 or more joints Symmetrical, affecting large joints, as well as fingers, cervical and temporomandibular joints	Chronic anterior uveitis	RF negative ANA positive ESR elevated
Seropositive polyarticular JIA	<10% of cases 9–12 years		Rheumatoid nodules	RF positive ESR elevated
Systemic JIA (Still's disease)	<10% of cases 2–4 years	Polyarthritis	Malaise, fever, salmon pink macular rash, lymphadenopathy, hepatosplenomegaly, serositis	RF negative, Elevated ESR Elevated acute phase proteins Anaemia Thrombocytosis

with arthritis affecting more than four joints with temporomandibular joint and finger involvement, which suggests a diagnosis of polyarticular JIA. Treatment mainly involves NSAIDs, steroids, and steroid-sparing agents (e.g. methotrexate).

Reactive arthritis is a sterile arthritis that occurs following an extra-articular infection, usually gastrointestinal or urogenital, and presents with the triad of arthritis, uveitis, and urethritis. Septic arthritis is an infection of a joint space (most commonly by *Staphylococcus aureus*) that can irreversibly and rapidly destroy a joint. The child will be acutely unwell and febrile with an acutely inflamed joint with a reduced range of movement.

4. C

Nappy rash (napkin dermatitis) is a form of irritant contact dermatitis in which the skin is damaged from exposure to irritants, such as urine, faeces, alcohol wipes, and friction. Other causes of nappy rash include *Candida* infection, impetigo, infantile seborrhoeic dermatitis, and atopic eczema. Parents or carers should be recommended high absorbency nappies, advised to change the nappy as soon as possible after soiling or wetting and use fragrance-free and alcohol-free wipes to clean the skin. If there is mild erythema and the child is asymptomatic, barrier protection can be applied at each nappy change to protect the skin. If the rash appears inflamed and is causing discomfort, children over 1 month of age can be prescribed a 7-day course of topical hydrocortisone 1% in addition to barrier protection. If nappy rash persists and bacterial infection is suspected or confirmed on a swab, a 7-day course of oral flucloxacillin should be considered. *Candida* infection characteristically causes satellite lesions and does not spare the skin folds. In such cases, barrier protection should be avoided and a topical imidazole cream (e.g. clotrimazole) should be prescribed.

5. B

Tuberous sclerosis is an autosomal dominant neurocutaneous disorder that is associated with abnormalities in multiple body systems:

- **Cutaneous:** Depigmented ash leaf shaped patches, shagreen patches (roughened patches of skin over the lumbar spine), angiofibromata in a butterfly distribution over the bridge of the nose and cheeks, and fibromas beneath the nail beds.
- **Neurological:** Infantile spasms, developmental delay, epilepsy, learning disabilities, subependymal nodules in the brain.
- **Cardiac:** Rhabdomyomas.
- **Eyes:** Retinal hamartomas.
- **Renal:** Angiomyolipoma, renal cell carcinoma.

Sturge–Weber syndrome is a sporadic disorder that manifests with a port-wine stain in the distribution of the ophthalmic division of the trigeminal nerve with associated intracranial lesions. Neurofibromatosis (NF) is an autosomal dominant condition that has two subtypes. NF type l is associated with café au lait spots, neurofibromas, optic gliomas, Lisch nodules, and sphenoid dysplasia. NF type ll is much rarer and is associated with schwannomas of the vestibulocochlear nerve (causing hearing loss), meningiomas, and spinal cord ependymomas. Tuberous sclerosis, Sturge–Weber syndrome, and NF are examples of neurocutaneous disorders. Rett syndrome is a sporadic disorder of brain development in which patients develop normally for the first 6–12 months, followed by a period of developmental regression. This is followed by a stage of plateau during which the child may show signs of improvement. Some patients will progress further to the final stage — deterioration of movement. This is characterised by scoliosis, muscle weakness, spasticity, and losing the ability to walk. Rett syndrome is caused by a mutation on the X chromosome and is typically fatal *in utero* in males.

6. B

Sudden infant death syndrome (SIDS) is the sudden, unexpected, and unexplained death of an apparently healthy infant under the age of 1 year. Most deaths happen during the first 6 months of life. Death usually occurs during sleep. The cause of SIDS is unknown, but risk factors are listed in the following table.

Infant	Environment	Parents
Age 1–6 months	Sleeping prone	Low income
Low birthweight and prematurity	Co-sleeping with parents	No maternal educational qualifications
Male	Overheating	Poor or overcrowded housing
Appeared ill in the previous 24 hours	Pillows	Maternal age <21 years
		Smoking or alcohol

SIDS is now rare due to the 'Back to Sleep' campaign which advised parents to place the infant on their back when they are being put to sleep. Parents should also be encouraged to place the infant with their feet at the end of the cot, keep their head uncovered, sleep in the same room for the first 6 months, use a firm, flat and waterproof mattress, and promote breastfeeding.

7. E

All children with an atypical urinary tract infection, irrespective of age, should receive an urgent ultrasound during the acute infection. Features of an atypical UTI include poor urine flow, abdominal or bladder mass, raised creatinine, sepsis, failure to respond to treatment with suitable antibiotics within 48 hours or infection with non-*E. coli* organisms. Children under 6 months old with recurrent UTI should also receive an urgent ultrasound scan during the acute infection.

A non-urgent ultrasound scan should be arranged within 6 weeks in children under the age of 6 months with a UTI and children over the age of 6 months with recurrent UTI. Dimercaptosuccinic acid scintigraphy (DMSA) should also be arranged within 4–6 months of the acute infection in all children aged under 3 years with atypical or recurrent UTI and all children aged 3 years and over with recurrent UTI. DMSA is a very sensitive scan that detects renal parenchymal defects. This patient is over 6 months old and has had recurrent UTIs so a non-urgent ultrasound scan within 6 weeks and a DMSA within 4–6 months should be arranged. The investigations and indications are outlined in the following table.

Test	Indications
US during acute infection	In all children with atypical infection, indicated by: • Poor urine flow • Abdominal or bladder mass • Raised creatinine • Sepsis • Failure to respond to antibiotics within 48 hours • Infection with non-*E. coli* organisms In children <6 months with recurrent UTI
US within 6 weeks	In children aged >6 months with recurrent UTI In children <6 months with first-time UTI
DMSA 4–6 months after acute infection	All children <3 years with atypical or recurrent UTI All children >3 years with recurrent UTI
MCUG	In children <6 months with atypical or recurrent UTI

8. D

Croup is a common upper respiratory tract condition that mainly occurs in babies and young children. It is usually caused by parainfluenza virus and presents with a seal-like barking cough and features of respiratory distress (e.g. stridor, sternal or intercostal recession). In severe cases, the child may appear agitated or lethargic. With any case of upper airway obstruction, the patient should be kept calm and placed on a parent's lap. All cases of croup, irrespective of severity should be treated with a single dose of 0.15 mg/kg oral dexamethasone immediately. This dose can be repeated after 12 hours if no improvement is observed. Although dexamethasone is the drug of choice, oral prednisolone and inhaled beclomethasone are possible alternatives. Moderate-to-severe croup with upper airway obstruction should be treated with high flow oxygen and nebulised adrenaline. Mild croup (barking cough with no other clinical features) can be treated as an outpatient. Croup of any greater severity requires admission for treatment. Croup typically has a relatively short course and patients should recover over about 48 hours.

9. E

In boys, the first sign of puberty is testicular enlargement (more than 4 mL), which is followed by the growth of pubic and axillary hair, deepening of the voice, acne, and development of a muscular physique. The growth spurt occurs about 18 months after the first signs of puberty. In girls, the first sign of puberty is development of palpable breast tissue, followed by pubic hair growth and a growth spurt. Menarche occurs about 2.5 years after the first signs of puberty. This child has precocious puberty defined as the onset of secondary sexual characteristics before the age of 8 years in girls and 9 years in boys. Causes of precocious puberty can be divided into gonadotrophin-dependent and gonadotrophin-independent. Gonadotrophin-dependent precious puberty occurs due to premature activation of the hypothalamic pituitary gonadal axis, resulting in an elevated follicle-stimulating hormone (FSH) and luteinising hormone (LH) level, and consonant puberty (i.e. following a normal sequence). This is very common in girls and is almost always idiopathic. However, it is much rarer in boys and often has a pathological cause, such as hydrocephalus, hypothyroidism or central nervous system abnormalities (e.g. hamartomas, irradiation, brain injury). Gonadotrophin-independent precocious puberty is caused by an excess of sex hormones from the gonads or adrenal glands. FSH and LH are low, and puberty is dissonant (i.e. following an abnormal sequence). Causes include adrenal tumours, congenital adrenal hyperplasia, ovarian/testicular tumours, and exogenous sex hormones. McCune–Albright syndrome is a genetic disorder associated with gonadotrophin-independent precocious puberty, café au lait spots and polyostotic fibrous dysplasia.

In boys, the cause of precious puberty may be identified on testicular examination. Bilateral enlargement suggests a gonadotrophin-dependent precocious puberty, whereas atrophic testes suggest a gonadotrophin-independent cause and a unilaterally enlarged testis suggests a gonadal tumour. The patient in this case has consonant puberty with bilaterally enlarged testes, suggesting a gonadotrophin-dependent cause, of which hypothalamic hamartoma is the only correct option.

10. D

Acute abdomen is defined as the rapid onset of severe abdominal pain that may indicate life-threatening intra-abdominal disease requiring urgent surgical intervention. Due to the age of the patient and recent onset of lower abdominal pain and nausea, a perforated appendix is the most likely underlying diagnosis. A large perforation results in generalised peritonitis, which manifests with high fever, diffuse abdominal pain, generalised tenderness, guarding, and absent bowel sounds. This patient requires an urgent exploratory laparotomy and appendicectomy.

An appendicular mass is another complication of appendicitis in which the inflamed appendix has an adherent covering of omentum and small bowel. These present similarly to appendicitis, but with a more gradual onset and examination may reveal a mass in the right iliac fossa. An appendicular abscess is a collection of pus from necrosis of tissue following perforation. Bowel obstruction would present with abdominal pain, absolute constipation, nausea and abdominal distension. In children, the most common cause of bowel obstruction is intussusception. Given this patient is 15 years of age, she is of reproductive age and a pregnancy test should be performed to exclude an ectopic pregnancy. This typically presents with unilateral lower abdominal pain, shoulder tip pain, amenorrhoea, and vaginal bleeding. An ectopic pregnancy can rupture leading to peritonitis.

11. A

Ringworm is a common skin infection that is often seen in primary care. The name is somewhat of a misnomer as it is, in fact, caused by a fungus (most commonly *Trichophyton*, *Microsporum*, and *Epidermophyton*). It is called 'ringworm' because of the ring-shaped (annular) red, scaly lesions that are characteristic of this disease. Mild infections, like the one described in this SBA, can be treated with topical antifungal creams such as terbinafine and clotrimazole. If there is a lot of inflammation, a hydrocortisone 1% cream can also be used.

Particularly severe or widespread infections will require systemic antifungals (usually oral terbinafine or itraconazole). If the ringworm infection involves the scalp (tinea capitis), systemic antifungals are generally recommended due to the difficulty of applying topical antifungals under the hair. As an extra precaution, any household pets of patients presenting with ringworm should receive treatment as it is a zoonotic disease. Conservative measures that should also be recommended include wearing loose-fitting clothing, washing affected areas daily, avoiding scratching, and frequently washing clothes and bed linen.

12. B

Atrioventricular septal defect (AVSD) is a congenital cardiac malformation in which the heart has a single large valve between both atria and ventricles. AVSD may be identified at the 20-week antenatal anomaly scan, but it may also present as a newborn with cyanosis or the development of heart failure after a few weeks of life. Typically, no murmur is heard with a complete AVSD, but an ECG may reveal left-axis deviation. AVSD is the most common heart murmur seen in children with Down syndrome.

Patients with atrial septal defects (ASD) are usually asymptomatic and will have an ejection systolic murmur best heard at the upper left sternal edge with a fixed widely split second heart sound. Ventricular septal defects (VSD) are the most common type of congenital heart defects. They are usually asymptomatic, but a loud pansystolic murmur may be heard at the lower left sternal edge with a quiet pulmonary second heart sound. Murmurs are typically louder for smaller defects, as the blood flow is more turbulent. Most small VSDs will close spontaneously, however large VSDs may lead to heart failure. Tricuspid atresia is the absence of the tricuspid valve leaving only a functional left ventricle and a small right ventricle. The child may be well at birth but become cyanosed or breathless with a pansystolic murmur. Interrupted aortic arch is a rare malformation in which there is no connection between the ascending and descending aorta. Cardiac output is dependent on a patent ductus arteriosus allowing blood from the pulmonary trunk to enter the descending aorta. A VSD is also usually present, in this condition, to allow mixing from between the left and right heart. Interrupted aortic arch is associated with genetic syndromes such as DiGeorge syndrome.

13. E

Hand, foot and mouth disease (HFMD) is a disease characterised by blisters on the hands and feet, vesicles in the mouth, palate and pharynx, and constitutional upset (fever, loss of appetite, irritability). HFMD is a self-limiting viral infection that is usually caused by an enterovirus (most commonly coxsackie A16 virus). It typically affects children under the age of 5 years. Management is largely supportive, for example, ensuring adequate fluid intake and using paracetamol or ibuprofen for symptomatic relief. Children do not need to be excluded from school and it should resolve spontaneously after 7–10 days.

Herpangina is similar to HFMD as it also causes painful mouth and throat ulcers and is caused by coxsackie A16 virus. The main difference is that the fever tends to be more prominent and the ulcers are only found on the soft palate, tonsils, uvula, and pharynx. Quinsy (peritonsilar abscess) is a rare and potentially serious complication of tonsillitis in which an abscess forms between one of the tonsils and the lateral wall of the pharynx. It presents with severe unilateral throat pain, fever, drooling, foul smelling breath, trismus, and changes to the voice. Molluscum contagiosum is a skin infection caused by a poxvirus which presents with clusters of umbilicated papules most often in the armpit, behind the knees, groin, and genital areas. Roseola infantum is caused by human herpes virus 6 and presents with a fever and malaise lasting 3–5 days, followed by an erythematous rash across the trunk and face. The rash may be seen on the soft palate (Nagayama spots).

14. C

Sickle cell disease is an autosomal recessive haemoglobinopathy caused by the presence of haemoglobin S (HbS). HbS forms due to a point mutation in codon 6 of the beta globin gene, which results in aggregation of Hb chains under low oxygen conditions. Sickle cells have a reduced lifespan and can become trapped in the microcirculation, resulting in blood vessel occlusion. This is responsible for the clinical manifestations of sickle cell disease:

- **Chronic haemolysis:** Anaemia, splenomegaly, gallstones, and aplastic crises (such as from parvovirus B19 infection).
- **Vaso-occlusive painful crises:** Dactylitis, acute chest syndrome, stroke, priapism, splenic sequestration (pooling of sickle cells in the spleen causing splenomegaly and hypotensive shock), autosplenectomy (splenic infarction leading to fibrosis), retinopathy, and renal dysfunction.

- **Infection:** Increased susceptibility to encapsulated organisms due to hyposplenism.
- **Long-term problems:** Short stature, delayed puberty, heart failure, psychosocial problems.

All children with painful crises should be admitted unless they have only mild or moderate pain and are apyrexial. An acute painful crisis should be treated as a medical emergency and patients should be given analgesia within 30 minutes and oxygen therapy if their saturation is 95% or lower. Children can be given regular paracetamol and NSAIDs in addition to an opioid. Corticosteroids are not recommended in uncomplicated acute painful crises. Children who have had recurrent hospital admissions for painful crises or acute chest syndrome may benefit from hydroxycarbamide, which works by increasing the concentration of foetal haemoglobin. It takes 6–8 weeks to cause a significant improvement, so is not appropriate in the acute setting. Children with sickle cell disease should be receiving prophylactic penicillin V, as well as folic acid and ensuring adequate nutrition and fluid intake, keeping up to date with immunisations and avoiding precipitants of painful crises (e.g. dehydration, cold and stress).

15. A

An episode of gastroenteritis followed by bloating and diarrhoea when a normal diet is reintroduced is suggestive of post-infectious irritable bowel syndrome. This most often occurs following gastroenteritis caused by *Campylobacter jejuni*. It tends to have a variable course but will usually settle over time and is associated with normal blood and stool tests. Transient lactose intolerance is another common complication of viral gastroenteritis that also presents with diarrhoea in the weeks after the initial infection has resolved.

Inflammatory bowel disease is increasing in incidence amongst children and adolescents and often presents with growth faltering, abdominal pain, diarrhoea (which may contain blood and mucus), lethargy, and extra-intestinal features (e.g. oral ulcers, uveitis, arthralgia, erythema nodosum, and pyoderma gangrenosum). Mesenteric adenitis is self-limiting inflammation of the mesenteric lymph nodes. It is associated with gastroenteritis (most commonly caused by *Yersinia enterocolitica*) and upper respiratory tract infections. It may present similarly to appendicitis with right iliac fossa pain. Giardiasis is a parasitic infection that causes chronic diarrhoea and faltering growth. Shigellosis is another cause of gastroenteritis and is particularly common in children. It causes diarrhoea (which may contain blood and mucus), fever and abdominal cramps, which usually resolves within a week.

16. B

The majority of children achieve day and night-time urinary continence by 3–4 years of age. Enuresis is involuntary urination which can be divided into primary (never achieved urinary continence) and secondary (loss of previously achieved urinary continence). The management of primary enuresis depends on the presence of daytime symptoms. All children with primary bedwetting and daytime symptoms (e.g. urgency, frequency) should be referred to secondary care or an enuresis clinic. For children with primary bedwetting without daytime symptoms, the management depends on age. All children (regardless of age) and their parents should be given advice on fluid intake, diet, and toileting patterns. For children younger than 5 years of age, patients should be reassured that it is not abnormal, and most children will become continent without treatment.

For children older than 5 years of age, the 1st line treatment option is an enuresis alarm with a positive reward system. An enuresis alarm senses wetness and triggers an alarm to wake the child with the aim of training them to recognise the need to urinate. If an alarm is offered, the child should be assessed after 4 weeks and if the child has responded, the alarm should be continued for a minimum of 14 consecutive dry nights. If the response is inadequate, desmopressin can be offered in combination with an alarm. Referral to secondary care or an enuresis clinic is only necessary if bedwetting has not responded to at least two complete courses of treatment with either an alarm or desmopressin.

17. D

This patient has presented with features suggestive of eczema herpeticum — a rare complication of eczema caused by disseminated herpes simplex virus infection. It tends to cause a fever and widespread blisters and punched-out erosions. It is a dermatological emergency and should be promptly treated with oral or IV aciclovir. If the eczema herpeticum is present around the eyes, an ophthalmological review should also be arranged.

Bacterial infection of eczema by *Staphylococcus aureus* and *Streptococcus pyogenes* may cause oozing from swollen, sore skin and a yellow crust may appear. Patients may also feel generally unwell with a fever. Varicella zoster virus causes chickenpox which presents with systemic upset and a widespread itchy vesicular rash. Parvovirus B19 causes slapped cheek syndrome (also known as fifth disease or erythema infectiosum). It causes a low-grade fever and a characteristic erythematous rash across the cheeks which has a 'slapped cheek' appearance. It is a self-limiting condition that gets better over the course of a few days.

18. C

Labial fusion is a benign condition in which the labia minora are joined together. It is common in girls under 7 years of age and usually resolves by puberty. It is not present at birth and usually develops at 1–2 years of age. The cause is unknown, but it may occur following inflammation (e.g. vulvovaginitis) or after trauma. Labial fusion rarely causes problems, but may cause local irritation, terminal dribbling, and increased risk of urinary tract infections. It is treated with topical oestrogen for 4–6 weeks, but this is only recommended if there are significant symptoms. Surgical separation may be considered if topical oestrogen is ineffective, the fusion is particularly thick and severe, or there is trapped urine which is causing terminal dribbling and vulval inflammation.

19. D

Congenital adrenal hyperplasia (CAH) is a group of autosomal recessive disorders of adrenal steroid biosynthesis. 90% of cases are caused by a deficiency of 21α-hydroxylase, an enzyme which is required for aldosterone and cortisol production. In the foetus, cortisol deficiency results in less negative feedback on the pituitary gland, which, in turn, results in increased ACTH production. ACTH has a stimulatory effect on adrenal androgen production. Excess androgens in girls results in virilisation (i.e. clitoral hypertrophy and labial fusion) and the development of ambiguous genitalia.

In boys, the penis may be enlarged, and the scrotum may be pigmented. The changes are less obvious in baby boys so they may present after a couple of weeks with a salt-losing crisis, caused by an aldosterone deficiency. The lack of aldosterone results in a high rate of urinary sodium loss (causing hyponatraemia). In the proximal convoluted tubule, sodium is secreted in exchange for hydrogen ions, resulting in a metabolic acidosis. Hyperkalaemia develops because aldosterone is responsible for potassium excretion and the cortisol deficiency results in hypoglycaemia. Infants with adrenal crises present with poor weight gain, vomiting, dehydration, and circulatory collapse, and respond rapidly to treatment with hydrocortisone, intravenous saline, and dextrose. The diagnosis of CAH can be made by measuring 17α-hydroxyprogesterone — a component of the adrenal steroid synthesis pathway which is raised due to excessive stimulation by ACTH.

20. E

Reactive arthritis is a sterile arthritis that occurs following an extra-articular infection, most commonly gastrointestinal (e.g. *Campylobacter*) or urogenital (e.g. *Chlamydia*). This patient has developed a triad of symptoms consistent with reactive arthritis: conjunctivitis, urethritis, and arthritis. These features generally appear within 1–3 weeks of infection and dysuria is usually the first symptom. This is followed by a transient asymmetric oligoarthritis affecting large joints, enthesitis (e.g. plantar fasciitis), and conjunctivitis. A small proportion of patients develop small hard nodules on the soles of the feet called keratoderma blenorrhagicum. Reactive arthritis belongs to the seronegative spondyloarthropathies — a group of rheumatologic disorders that are rheumatoid factor negative and associated with HLA-B27.

Systemic lupus erythematosus (SLE) is rare in children and is more likely to present in adolescent females. The features of SLE can be remembered using the mnemonic **SOAP BRAIN MD**: **S**erositis, **O**ral ulcers, **A**rthritis, **P**hotosensitivity, **B**lood disorders (e.g. haemolytic anaemia), **R**enal disease (e.g. proteinuria, haematuria), **A**NA positive, **I**mmunological features (e.g. anti-dsDNA), **N**eurologic disease (e.g. seizures, psychosis), **M**alar rash, and **D**iscoid rash. Juvenile idiopathic arthritis is persistent joint swelling (more than 6 weeks) presenting before 16 years of age in the absence of infection or any other cause. Kawasaki disease is a medium vessel vasculitis mainly affecting children under 5 years old. It presents with a fever lasting more than 5 days, conjunctivitis, mucous membrane changes, cervical lymphadenopathy, and erythema and oedema of the hands and feet. Juvenile dermatomyositis presents with progressive muscle weakness and a facial rash.

21. D

If a child has a febrile seizure, parents or carers should be advised to record the duration of the seizure, protect the child from injury during the seizure, check that the airway is patent and place the child in the recovery position once the seizure has terminated. If tonic–clonic movements last for more than 5 minutes, emergency benzodiazepine rescue medication (buccal midazolam or rectal diazepam) should be administered. If the seizure persists for more than 5 minutes after the first dose of benzodiazepine, an ambulance should be called, and rescue therapy can be repeated.

The child should not be placed in the recovery position until the seizure has stopped because this would involve a degree of physical restraint which could lead to injury. Prophylactic antipyretics at the onset of the fever are not recommended as this does not prevent recurrence of febrile seizures. It would also be unsafe to attempt to administer an oral medication in a seizing child because of the risk of aspiration.

22. B

Congenital diaphragmatic hernia describes herniation of the abdominal contents through the posterolateral foramen of the diaphragm which occurs due to incomplete formation of the diaphragm. Compression of the lungs by the herniated viscera impedes normal lung development resulting in pulmonary hypoplasia. Newborns will present with respiratory distress and failure to respond to resuscitation. Heart sounds may be displaced with absent air entry and audible bowel sounds in the chest. Patients may also have a barrel-shaped chest and a scaphoid abdomen. A chest X-ray will show abdominal contents and poorly aerated lungs in the ipsilateral hemithorax with mediastinal shift. Most cases are identified at antenatal ultrasound scans. Once diagnosed, patients should be intubated and ventilated, and a nasogastric tube should be inserted to aspirate the gastrointestinal contents and ease the compression. Definitive treatment is surgical.

Neonatal pneumothorax may occur with ventilation and the presentation varies from asymptomatic to life-threatening respiratory distress. Neonatal pneumonia typically occurs with prolonged rupture of membranes, chorio-amnionitis or prematurity and presents with respiratory distress, cough, neutropenia, and temperature instability. Hypoxic ischaemic encephalopathy is neonatal brain damage that occurs due to a significant hypoxic event during labour or delivery. Oesophageal atresia is a congenital malformation in which the oesophagus is a blind-ended pouch that fails to reach the stomach. In most cases, there is a fistula between the distal oesophagus and trachea, and infants typically present with choking or coughing during feeds.

23. B

Drowsiness should always be taken seriously as it may be a sign of major underlying pathology. The increased respiratory rate may lead clinicians to consider sepsis secondary to a chest infection, however, the CXR findings and normal vital signs suggest that it is unlikely. The CXR incidentally noticed two posterior rib fractures, which is unusual in a child of any age. This finding should raise suspicion of non-accidental injury as grabbing the child can lead to such rib fractures. Furthermore, the failure to vaccinate the child may suggest that the family may not have been interacting with health services appropriately.

The constellation of symptoms caused by vigorously shaking a baby or small child is sometimes referred to as 'shaken baby syndrome'. Features include posterior rib fractures, encephalopathy (usually presenting with drowsiness) due to a subdural haematoma, and retinal haemorrhages. If NAI is suspected, the patient should be admitted, and the safeguarding team should be informed. Patients should undergo a panel of investigations to identify the aforementioned manifestations of vigorous shaking. A CT head scan should be requested to identify a subdural haemorrhage, fundoscopy to identify retinal haemorrhages, and a skeletal survey to identify any other broken bones. If the predominant presenting feature is bruising of unknown origin, a coagulation screen, bone profile, and full blood count should be performed to identify any haematological causes such as leukaemia, thrombocytopaenia, clotting defects, and vitamin D deficiency.

24. E

Glucose-6-phosphate dehydrogenase deficiency (G6PD) is an X-linked recessive enzyme defect which results in a glutathione deficiency resulting in red cells that are vulnerable to oxidative stress. When exposed to oxidants, there is an acute intravascular haemolytic crisis that presents with fever, malaise, dark urine, jaundice, and a rapidly declining haemoglobin. Infection is the most common precipitant, but others include anti-malarial agents (e.g. primaquine), antibiotics (e.g. sulphonamides), analgesics (e.g. aspirin), and chemicals (e.g. fava beans). As well as acute crises, G6PD deficiency is the most common cause of neonatal jaundice worldwide. During a haemolytic crisis, blood tests will reveal anaemia, reticulocytosis, hyperbilirubinaemia, raised LDH, reduced haptoglobins, and haemoglobinuria. A blood film may show bite cells, blister cells, and Heinz bodies. Between haemolytic crises, patients are asymptomatic with a normal blood film and biochemistry. A diagnosis can be made with an enzyme assay 2–3 months following a crisis.

Pyruvate kinase deficiency is an autosomal recessive enzyme defect that causes a chronic haemolytic anaemia and a blood film will typically reveal echinocytes. Hereditary spherocytosis is an autosomal dominant membrane defect that results in extravascular haemolysis (splenomegaly), jaundice and gallstones, and a blood film will show spherocytes (hyperchromic spherical red cells). Parvovirus B19 infection and Diamond–Blackfan anaemia are both causes of red cell aplasia due to bone marrow failure. This therefore produces a low reticulocyte count. Diamond–Blackfan anaemia is an autosomal dominant disorder which presents with anaemia at 2–3 months and is associated physical abnormalities, such as microcephaly, absent thumbs, and cleft palate.

25. A

This child appears to have gastro-oesophageal reflux. It is a common condition characterised by frequent vomiting after feeds which can affect growth. It is thought to occur due to functional immaturity of the lower oesophageal sphincter. The vast majority of babies with symptoms of gastro-oesophageal reflux will not need treatment, however, in the presence of faltering growth, treatment should be considered. In breastfed infants, a breastfeeding assessment should be carried out after which alginate therapy should be trialled for 1–2 weeks. Alginates are oral agents that precipitate and thicken once they enter the stomach. Thickening the stomach contents makes regurgitation less likely. Other treatment options if alginate therapy is unsuccessful include proton pump inhibitors (e.g. omeprazole) and histamine antagonists (e.g. ranitidine). In formula-fed infants, initial management involves trialling smaller, more frequent feeds, a trial of thickened formula and alginate therapy. In children with severe disease, admission for enteral feeding and Nissen fundoplication may be considered. It is important to take a holistic approach to managing these patients as there may be other factors contributing to the clinical situation. For example, the mental and physical wellbeing of the mother should be assessed to ensure adequate breast milk production and other causes of failure to thrive (e.g. malabsorption) should be considered.

The management of gastro-oesophageal reflux in children is summarised in the following RevChart.

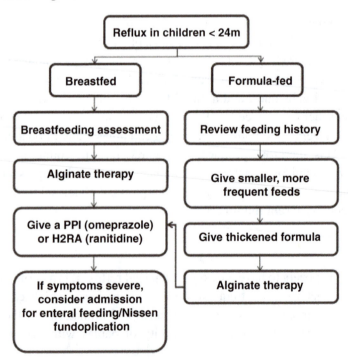

26. B

Most murmurs heard in children are innocent murmurs, which are caused by physiological changes leading to increased flow, as opposed to structural heart defects. It can be difficult to distinguish innocent murmurs from murmurs resulting from congenital cardiac defects, however, there are four hallmarks of innocent murmurs which can be remembered as the 4 **S**'s:

- A**S**ymptomatic
- **S**ystolic or throughout systole and diastole (i.e. never diastolic only)
- **S**oft blowing murmur
- Loudest at left **S**ternal edge

Innocent murmurs also do not radiate, and no added sounds will be heard. Furthermore, as the murmur is primarily caused by increased flow, it may be heard best when the child is ill and, therefore, tachycardic. Murmurs may also change with position (e.g. squatting may make a murmur disappear). In some patients, especially newborns, distinguishing innocent murmurs may require further investigations, such as ECG and CXR.

27. C

The development of children should be assessed whenever the child has contact with healthcare, as early intervention with developmental delays can help ameliorate their long-term impact. The causes of developmental delay vary depending on the type of delay, for example, a delay in hearing, speech, and language may be due to a hearing impairment or having a bilingual household, whereas a delay in gross motor function may be due to neuromuscular problems such as muscular dystrophy. Development is assessed using median age (age at which half of a population of children will develop a certain skill) and limit age (age by which 95% of the population of children would have developed a certain skill). Passing a limit age is an indication for further investigation.

There are four main domains of childhood development and the key median and limit ages are listed in the following table.

Domain	Skill	Median age	Limit age
Gross motor	Control of head	6–8 weeks	4 months
	Sits unsupported	6–8 months	9 months
	Stands independently	10 months	12 months
	Walks independently	12 months	18 months
Vision and fine motor	Fixes and follows	6 weeks	3 months
	Reaches for objects	4 months	6 months
	Transfers between hands	7 months	9 months
	Mature pincer grip	10 months	12 months
Social, emotional and behavioural	Smiles	6 weeks	8 weeks
	Feeds with spoon	15 months	18 months
	Symbolic play	18 months	2.5 years
	Interactive play	2.5 years	3.5 years
Hearing, speech and language	Babbles	4 months	8 months
	Says 'mama' and 'dada'	10 months	18 months
	Says 6 words with meaning	18 months	2.5 years
	Joins words	2 years	3.5 years

The child in this question is normal in all domains except hearing, speech, and language, in which she has passed the limit age for saying 6 words with meaning (2.5 years).

28. D

Scarlet fever is an infectious disease caused by toxin-producing strains of *Streptococcus pyogenes* (Group A *streptococcus*). The throat is usually the primary site of infection, causing a pharyngitis. The first clinical features are non-specific, such as a sore throat, fever, and flu-like symptoms. This is followed by 12–48 hours later by a blanching rash, which starts on the abdomen and spreads to the neck and limbs. The rash is red and punctate with a rough, sandpaper-like texture. Examination may reveal a strawberry tongue (initially with a white coat and enlarged papillae, followed by a beefy red appearance), cervical lymphadenopathy, pharyngitis, and red macules on the palate.

Prompt antibiotic treatment with a 10-day course of phenoxymethylpenicillin (penicillin V) is required. Symptomatic treatment with simple analgesia, adequate fluid intake, and rest should be recommended. Scarlet fever is a notifiable disease so the local Health Protection Unit should be informed. As it is highly contagious, children should avoid nursery or school until 24 hours after commencing antibiotics. Symptoms usually resolve within 1 week. Hospital admission should be considered in patients at increased risk of complications (e.g. pre-existing valvular heart disease) or if they have already developed complications (e.g. streptococcal glomerulonephritis). Kawasaki disease is an important differential for scarlet fever and is treated with high-dose aspirin and IVIG.

29. D

Cystic fibrosis is an autosomal recessive condition which arises due to a mutation in the cystic fibrosis transmembrane conductance regulator (CFTR), a chloride channel that is responsible for efflux of chloride ions. This process is important in allowing water to enter secretions thus making them less viscid. A dysfunctional CFTR results in thickened secretions in various sites across the body, most importantly, the respiratory tract and gastrointestinal tract. Cystic fibrosis is typically diagnosed during the heel prick test, which measures levels of serum immune reactive trypsinogen and uses genetic analysis of common CFTR mutations. As this child was born outside the UK, it is likely that this screening test was unavailable at the time of his birth. A delay in the passage of meconium within the first 24 hours of life is suggestive of cystic fibrosis. If undiagnosed at birth, children may present with faltering growth, recurrent chest infections, rectal prolapse, and nasal polyps. Later complications of cystic fibrosis include bronchiectasis, diabetes mellitus, cirrhosis, and sterility in males. A summary of the systems affected, main features, and treatment options are shown in the following table.

System	Features	Treatment
Respiratory	Chronic cough, recurrent chest infections	Physiotherapy Mucoactive agents Antibiotic prophylaxis
Gastrointestinal	Pancreatic exocrine insufficiency Malabsorption	Vitamin supplementation High-calorie diet

(Continued)

(*Continued*)

System	Features	Treatment
Infection	Recurrent infections	Antibiotic prophylaxis Vaccination
Psychiatric	Depression Anxiety	Child and adolescent mental health services

30. C

Anaphylaxis should be suspected in cases of sudden-onset difficulty breathing with rapid progression of the symptoms. Other symptoms include stridor, wheeze, cyanosis, drowsiness, and urticaria. Those with a low blood pressure should be positioned lying flat with their legs elevated and administer 1:1000 intramuscular adrenaline (0–6 years: 0.15 mL; 6–12 years: 0.3 mL; 12+ years: 0.5 mL). They are then re-assessed after 5 minutes and IM adrenaline can be repeated at 5-minute intervals until there has been an adequate response. Patients should also be put on high-flow oxygen and IV access should be established to give a rapid fluid challenge (20 mL/kg). The aspects of management of anaphylaxis can be remembered using the mnemonic **FLACOS** — **F**luids, **L**egs elevated, **A**drenaline, **C**hlorphenamine, **O**xygen, and **S**albutamol.

Nebulised salbutamol or ipratropium is considered if the child is wheezy or a known asthmatic. Following emergency treatment, the child should be referred to an allergy clinic and provided with two adrenaline auto-injectors. Oral prednisolone can be given in mild cases of anaphylaxis but is not safe if the swallow is impaired (e.g. in a drowsy patient) and nebulised adrenaline is used to treat severe croup.

Paediatrics: Paper 3

Questions

1. A 4-year-old girl presents to A&E with a 7-day history of fever, rash, and sore eyes. On examination, there is a widespread maculopapular rash, the oral mucosa appears inflamed and cervical lymph nodes are enlarged. What is the most likely underlying diagnosis?

    A Rheumatic fever
    B Systemic juvenile idiopathic arthritis
    C Scarlet fever
    D Macrophage activation syndrome
    E Kawasaki disease

2. A 2-year-old boy presents with a third episode of intussusception. He is complaining of abdominal pain and has been refusing food for the last day. The pain tends to come and go in waves and an ultrasound scan confirm a diagnosis of intussusception. Which of the following would be most appropriate to identify the cause of recurrent intussusception?

    A Abdominal X-ray
    B Colonoscopy
    C Oesophago-gastro-duodenoscopy
    D Technetium-99m Scan
    E MIBG Scan

3. An 11-year-old boy presents with a limp that has got progressively worse over the past 4 weeks. He complains of some left-sided knee pain when walking and, on examination, there is restricted abduction and internal rotation of the left hip. He has a past medical history of hypothyroidism and his BMI is in the 95th centile. What is the most likely diagnosis?

    A Perthes disease
    B Slipped capital femoral epiphysis
    C Juvenile idiopathic arthritis
    D Transient synovitis
    E Osgood–Schlatter disease

4. A 6-year-old girl from the Philippines presents to A&E with severe breathing difficulties. She has a high fever and her breathing has deteriorated rapidly over the past 3 hours. On examination, she is sat upright on the examination couch and she is drooling from her mouth. What is the most appropriate first step to take?

    A Transfer to ITU
    B Examine the throat for an obstruction
    C Administer oral benzylpenicillin
    D Administer salbutamol inhaler through a spacer
    E Administer intramuscular adrenaline

5. A 15-year-old boy from Turkey presents complaining of general tiredness and difficulty concentrating in school. He is otherwise well and has no significant past medical history. A blood film shows microcytic and hypochromic red cells. His blood test results are shown below:

Haemoglobin: 120 g/L (130–175)
Mean cell volume: 65 fL (80–96)
Ferritin: 120 ug/L (12–200)

What is the most likely diagnosis?

    A Iron deficiency anaemia
    B Beta thalassaemia major

    C Beta thalassaemia trait
    D Sickle cell trait
    E Haemoglobin Barts

6. A 5-month-old boy has had continuous struggles feeding and seems to be relatively drowsy and inactive compared to others his age. He is also noted as being on the 3rd centile for length. On examination, he has a large tongue and a small umbilical hernia. What is the most likely underlying diagnosis?

    A Constitutional growth delay
    B Growth hormone deficiency
    C Congenital hypothyroidism
    D Cushing syndrome
    E Prader–Willi syndrome

7. Which of the following physiological changes in the circulatory system occurs immediately after birth?

    A Closure of the ductus arteriosus
    B Opening of the foramen ovale
    C Increase in venous return to the right atrium
    D Increase in left atrial pressure
    E Increase in pulmonary resistance

8. An 8-year-old girl is being resuscitated by a pedestrian following a car accident. The airway is patent, and 5 rescue breaths are given. Her breathing is irregular, and her pulse is 36 bpm. What is the next most step in resuscitating her?

    A Repeat 5 rescue breaths
    B Perform 15 chest compressions
    C Give 2 rescue breaths
    D Place the child in the recovery position
    E Administer intramuscular adrenaline

9. A 16-year-old girl has developed a sore throat and swallowing discomfort. On examination, there are 10–20 tender erythematous nodules on both shins measuring 2–5 cm in diameter. What is this dermatological phenomenon?

   A Erythema nodusum
   B Erythema multiforme
   C Guttate psoriasis
   D Erythema migrans
   E Erythema marginatum

10. An 8-year-old girl has a BMI that is on the 95th centile for her age. She does not complain of any joint pain or sleep apnoea. Her mother has heard about an obesity prevention drug called *Orlistat* and would like to know more about whether it would benefit her daughter. How should she be advised?

    A It is never recommended in children
    B It is generally not recommended in children under 12 years old
    C It is only recommended in children following bariatric surgery
    D It is only recommended in children with a BMI above the 98th percentile
    E It is only recommended in children with a BMI above the 91st percentile

11. A 9-year-old boy presents to A&E with scrotal pain that has been getting worse over the last 3 days. On examination, there is tenderness over the upper pole of the right testicle, the cremasteric reflex is positive and a blue dot is visible on the scrotum. What is the most likely diagnosis?

    A Hydrocele
    B Epdidymitis

C Varicocele

D Hydatid torsion

E Testicular torsion

12. A 6-year-old boy, who was diagnosed with asthma 2 years ago, has been experiencing 4 episodes of breathlessness and night time coughing per week over the last 3 months. He is currently using a salbutamol reliever inhaler and a paediatric low dose budesonide preventer inhaler. What is the most appropriate next step in his management?

A Switch to moderate dose budesonide

B Change to maintenance and reliever therapy

C Add leukotriene receptor antagonist

D Add omalizumab

E Add oral steroids

13. A 7-year-old boy is referred to paediatrics after complaints from teachers about episodes of staring blankly into space during which he is unresponsive. His eyelids may flicker, and he appears confused after these episodes. They last up to 15 seconds and occur between 10 and 20 times per day. An EEG shows fast generalised 3 Hz spike and wave patterns. What is the most likely diagnosis?

A Infantile spasms

B Juvenile myoclonic epilepsy

C Lennox–Gastaut syndrome

D Childhood absence epilepsy

E Childhood epilepsy with centro-temporal spikes

14. A 9-year-old girl presents with a rash on both cheeks. She has been off school for 5 days with a fever, runny nose, and diarrhoea, but the rash was first noticed yesterday. On examination, there is an erythematous maculopapular rash on the face, trunk, and back. What is the most likely diagnosis?

    A Measles
    B Rubella
    C Mumps
    D Infectious mononucleosis
    E Erythema infectiosum

15. A 3-year-old boy has developed a red rash over his buttocks and some vague abdominal pain. He has recently been recovering from a cough and a cold before these symptoms started. His vital signs are shown below:

Temperature: 37.3°C
Blood pressure: 132/96 mm Hg
Heart rate: 102 bpm
Respiratory rate: 24 breaths/min
SaO_2: 98% on air
Urine dipstick: + protein ++ blood

What is the most likely diagnosis?

    A Meningococcal sepsis
    B Idiopathic thrombocytopaenic purpura
    C Thrombotic thrombocytopaenic purpura
    D Haemophilia
    E Henoch–Schonlein purpura

16. A 2-year-old girl is brought to see her GP after some breast tissue growth was noticed by her parents. This was first noticed 6 months ago, and it has not changed in appearance since. She has not had a growth spurt, grown pubic hair, or developed acne. What is the most appropriate management option?

    A Measure LH, FSH, and oestradiol
    B Arrange chromosomal karyotyping
    C Reassure and arrange follow up
    D Prescribe gonadotrophin releasing hormone analogue therapy
    E Arrange an MRI head

17. What is the term used to describe a congenital deformity of the feet of a newborn in which the forefoot is adducted with a hindfoot varus?

    A Pes cavus
    B Pes planus
    C Vertical talus
    D Talipes equinovarus
    E Positional talipes

18. A 3-week-old boy has been vomiting after every feed. The vomiting has gradually increased in frequency and force, recently becoming projectile. The vomit is not bilious, and he usually wants to continue feeding afterwards. Given the most likely diagnosis, which of the following examination findings would you expect to find?

    A Dystonic neck movements and arching of the back
    B Drawing up of the knees
    C Palpation over the left iliac fossa cause pain in the right iliac fossa
    D A sausage-shaped abdominal mass is palpable
    E A peristalsis wave moving from left to right is visible after feeding

19. An 18-month-old boy is brought to see his GP after he has developed dry, flaky skin across his torso and on his cheeks. This has been present for about 1 month and he often tries to itch his torso through his clothes. He has also had difficulty sleeping. On examination, the skin on his torso appears dry with some slightly erythematous areas. A management plan of frequent emollient use and a mild potency steroid cream to use once per day until the inflammation settles is agreed upon with his father. Which of the following creams would be appropriate in this scenario?

    A Hydrocortisone 1%
    B Betamethasone valerate 0.025%
    C Clobetasone butyrate 0.05%

    D Clobetasol proprionate 0.1%

    E Mometasone furoate 0.1%

20. On neonatal examination, a baby is noted to have a prominent occiput, micrognathia, rocker-bottom feet, overlapping fingers, and dysplastic ears. What is the most likely diagnosis?

    A Patau syndrome

    B Pierre Robin sequence

    C Edwards syndrome

    D Foetal alcohol syndrome

    E Down syndrome

21. A 15-year-old girl presents to the GP with a 7-day history of a sore throat which has not improved. She returned from a festival last week and has since been feeling generally unwell with a fever and headache. On examination, there is cervical lymphadenopathy, tonsillar enlargement, and splenomegaly. A blood film shows 25% atypical lymphocytes. How should this patient be managed?

    A Admit to hospital

    B Prescribe oral amoxicillin and advise that school absence is not necessary

    C Prescribe clarithromycin and advise school absence for 48 hours after commencing treatment

    D Advise on bed rest, pain relief and fluids and that school absence is not necessary

    E Prescribe penicillin V and advise school absence for 24 hours after commencing treatment

22. A 1-week-old boy is brought to the ambulatory care centre by his father who claims that he often chokes and struggles to breathe when he is feeding. He explains that he often 'turns blue' which resolves when he starts to cry. He does not have fever or other flu-like symptoms. What is the most likely diagnosis?

A Tetralogy of Fallot
B Peritonsillar abscess
C Choanal atresia
D Laryngomalacia
E Transposition of the great arteries

23. A 1-day-old neonate is due to have his first baby check. On examination, it is noted that there is an opening on the ventral surface of his penis. A urethral meatus cannot be seen at the tip of the penis. He has produced several wet nappies since birth, but his parents have not yet noticed any abnormalities with the stream. What is the most likely diagnosis?

A Phimosis
B Paraphimosis
C Hypospadias
D Labial adhesion
E Balanoposthitis

24. A 10-month old girl is seen in the outpatient clinic regarding her poor growth. Her weight has fallen from the 54th centile to the 32nd centile. This began after she was weaned from breast milk to solids at the age of 6 months. On examination, the child is pale with some evidence of buttock wasting. She has frequent loose stools but feeds well. What is the most likely diagnosis?

A Coeliac disease
B Cows' milk protein allergy
C Gastroenteritis
D Giardiasis
E Inflammatory bowel disease

25. An 8-year-old boy is rushed into A&E by the paramedics. He has been seizing for 15 minutes and has already received one dose of buccal midazolam in the ambulance. 15 L/min of oxygen is given

through a non-rebreather mask and intravenous access is established. What is the next best step in the management of this child?

    A Repeat buccal midazolam
    B Rectal diazepam
    C IV lorazepam
    D IV phenytoin
    E Intubate and ventilate and IV thiopental sodium

26. A 1-day-old baby boy with bilious vomiting and abdominal disten-tion is found to have a 'double bubble sign' on an abdominal radio-graph. He also has epicanthal folds, up-slanting palpebral fissures, and a single palmar crease. What is the most likely diagnosis?

    A Biliary atresia
    B Gastroschisis
    C Necrotising enterocolitis
    D Intestinal malrotation
    E Duodenal atresia

27. A 6-year-old girl presents with a 2-day history of a severely itchy scalp. There has been a recent outbreak of nits in her primary school and, on examination, lice can be seen on the nape of the neck and there are red spots on the skin. How can this condition be managed?

    A Attempt wet combing and advise not to attend school until lice are undetectable
    B Attempt wet combing and advise that it is safe to attend school
    C Treat with dimeticone 4% lotion and advise not to attend school until lice are undetectable
    D Treat with dimeticone 4% lotion and advise that it is safe to attend school
    E Treat with permethrin 5% cream and advise to decontaminate all bedding and clothes

28. Which of the following is associated with cerebral palsy?

    A Dry mouth
    B Chronic diarrhoea
    C Hyperacusis
    D Sleep disturbance
    E Macroglossia

29. A 7-year-old boy presents to A&E with sudden-onset watery diarrhoea and vomiting. On examination, he has dry mucous membranes and reduced skin turgor. His hands feel warm with strong peripheral pulses and a capillary refill time of 2 seconds. His observations are listed in the following:

    Heart rate: 115 bpm
    Blood pressure: 105/70 mm Hg
    Respiratory rate: 24 breaths/min
    Temperature: 37.0°C

    Which of the following best describes this patient's hydration status?

    A No clinically detectable dehydration
    B Clinical dehydration
    C Clinical shock
    D Hypernatraemic dehydration
    E Impossible to tell without weight

30. A 5-year-old boy has had some difficulty breathing and a fever of 39°C. On examination, there is marked chest recession, reduced air entry, and coarse crackles in the left lower lobe with peripheral cyanosis. His vital signs are shown in the following:

    Heart rate: 142 bpm
    Respiratory rate: 46 breaths/min
    Temperature: 38.7°C
    Blood pressure: 104/64 mm Hg
    Oxygen saturation: 91% on air

What is the most appropriate initial management option?

A Call an ambulance and administer oxygen
B Prescribe amoxicillin
C Prescribe amoxicillin and erythromycin
D Reassure and discharge
E Prescribe dexamethasone

Answers

1. E

Kawasaki disease is a small vessel vasculitis that tends to affect children under 5 years old. It is diagnosed clinically in children with a fever that has lasted 5 days or longer and who have four of the following five features:

1. Bilateral non-exudative conjunctivitis
2. Change in mucous membranes of the upper respiratory tract (such as dry cracked lips or strawberry tongue)
3. Changes in the extremities (such as oedema, erythema, or desquamation)
4. Polymorphous rash
5. Cervical lymphadenopathy

This can be remembered using the mnemonic **CRASH and Burn** — **C**onjunctivitis, **R**ash, **A**denopathy, **S**trawberry tongue, involvement of **H**ands and feet and fever (**Burn**). Although rare, Kawasaki disease is an important diagnosis to consider because coronary artery aneurysms are a potentially life-threatening complication that require early detection with an echocardiogram. It is treated with prompt intravenous immunoglobulin within 10 days of the onset of symptoms and high-dose aspirin.

Scarlet fever presents similarly to Kawasaki disease, however, the main differences are the presence of cracked lips and non-suppurative conjunctivitis in Kawasaki disease. Rheumatic fever is a systemic disease occurring after a group A streptococcal throat infection due to molecular mimicry. A diagnosis is made if two of the following five 'Jones' criteria are present: carditis, polyarthritis, chorea, subcutaneous nodules and Sydenham chorea. Systemic juvenile idiopathic arthritis (JIA) causes a polyarthritis accompanied by a salmon pink macular rash, hepatosplenomegaly, fever, and serositis. Macrophage activation syndrome describes excessive expansion of T lymphocytes and macrophages and is a life-threatening complication of any rheumatic disease (including systemic JIA and Kawasaki disease), which has three cardinal features — cytopenia, liver dysfunction, and coagulopathy.

2. D

Recurrent intussusception should be investigated further to identify possible pathological lead points that leads to invagination of the bowel. A Meckel's diverticulum is a vestigial remnant of the omphalomesenteric duct. Its key features can be remembered as the 'rule of 2s' — present in 2% of the population, usually presents under the age of 2 years, lies within 2 feet of the ileo-caecal valve, and roughly 2 inches in length. Many cases will be asymptomatic, but they can cause recurrent intussusception and rectal bleeding. It often contains ectopic gastric mucosa and can, therefore, be identified using a technetium-99m scan which is a form of nuclear imaging that highlights gastric mucosa. An area of ectopic gastric mucosa will be seen in patients with Meckel's diverticulum. If symptomatic, a Meckel's diverticulum may be surgically removed.

An abdominal X-ray may be useful in cases of bowel obstruction but is unlikely to show the underlying defect giving rise to the obstruction. Modes of endoscopy such as colonoscopy and oesophago-gastro-duodenoscopy should be avoided except under specialist advice as they are distressing to young children. A MIBG scan is another type of nuclear scan which is useful for identifying phaeochomocytomas.

3. B

Slipped capital femoral epiphysis (SCFE) is posteroinferior displacement of the epiphysis of the femoral head, which places the femoral head at risk of avascular necrosis. It usually presents insidiously with a limp or hip pain (that may be referred to the knee) but may present acutely after trauma. Examination may find pain on abduction and internal rotation of the hip. Perthes disease is a similar condition characterised by avascular necrosis of the capital femoral epiphysis. The main difference is that SCFE is more likely to occur in 10–15-year-old children, whereas Perthes disease tends to occur in 5–10-year-old children. SCFE is also associated with obesity and endocrine abnormalities, such as hypothyroidism, whereas Perthes disease is associated with short stature and hyperactivity. Furthermore, SCFE is more likely to be bilateral.

A summary of bone and joint conditions is children is outlined in the following table.

Condition	Key features
Developmental dysplasia of the hip (DDH)	Positive Barlow and Ortolani test at neonatal screening If missed, presents in infancy with a waddling gait, leg length discrepancy, asymmetrical skin folds, and limited hip abduction Risk Factors: family history, breech birth, prematurity, oligohydramnios, multiple pregnancy, and female gender
Transient synovitis (irritable hip)	Peak incidence in 2–12 year olds and more common in boys The most common cause of acute hip pain in children Presents with pain or limp following a viral infection without pain at rest Patients are afebrile and appear well
Septic arthritis	Peak incidence in <4 year olds and more common in boys Presents with acute onset joint pain which is present at rest Most commonly affects the hip The hip is held flexed and the child appears very unwell
Perthes disease	Peak incidence in 5–10 year olds and more common in boys Presents with insidious onset of limp, hip or knee pain and pain on internal rotation and abduction Associated with hyperactivity and short stature
Slipped capital femoral epiphysis	Peak incidence in 10–15 year olds and more common in boys Presents with insidious or acute onset limp, hip or knee pain and pain on internal rotation and abduction Associated with obesity and endocrine abnormalities (e.g. hypothyroidism, hypogonadism, etc.)
Osgood–Schlatter disease	Peak incidence in 10–15 year olds and more common in boys Presents with knee pain after exercise and localised tenderness and swelling over the tibial tuberosity Associated with physical activity
Chondromalacia patellae	Peak incidence in 15–35 year olds and more common girls Presents with knee pain when standing up from sitting and walking up stairs Associated with physical activity
Juvenile idiopathic arthritis	Peak incidence in 10–15 year olds and more common girls Presents with persistent joint swelling (>6 weeks) Please refer to **Paediatrics Paper 2 Explanation 3** for more information

4. A

Acute Epiglottitis is a potentially life-threatening condition in which there is a rapid swelling of the epiglottis caused by *Haemophilus influenzae* type b. Children will typically present acutely unwell with a high fever and a painful throat that limits their ability to speak or swallow. There may be a soft stridor and the child may be sitting upright, immobile and drooling from the mouth. Fortunately, acute epiglottitis has become very rare after the introduction of the *Haemophilus influenzae* type b vaccine. Patients with suspected acute epiglottitis should be made as comfortable as possible and urgently transferred to the intensive care unit where their airway should be secured. Both the anaesthetics and ENT teams should be contacted as failure to secure the airway with intubation may require a surgical airway. A blood culture should be taken and IV empirical antibiotics (e.g. ceftriaxone) should be commenced. With treatment, most children will recover within 2–3 days.

Examination of the throat should generally be avoided in children with stridor as it could precipitate total obstruction of the airway. It should only be considered in the presence of an anaesthetist capable of rapidly intubating the patient if necessary. A salbutamol inhaler will not be effective in this situation as the obstruction is in the upper airway and it risks upsetting the child, potentially resulting in respiratory arrest. IM adrenaline is only used in cases of airway obstruction caused by anaphylaxis. However, nebulised adrenaline may be a useful adjunct to help relieve the obstruction.

5. C

The blood test results show a microcytic anaemia — the causes of which can be remembered via the mnemonic **TAILS**: Thalassaemia, Anaemia of chronic disease, Iron deficiency, Lead poisoning and Sideroblastic anaemia. Thalassaemia is an autosomal recessive haemoglobinopathy caused by a mutation in the alpha-globin or beta-globin gene. It is particularly prevalent in people of Mediterranean and Middle Eastern origin. There are two main types of beta thalassaemia:

- **Beta thalassaemia major:** Home zygous form where there is no beta chain production and an absolute deficiency of HbA.

Children become profoundly anaemic at 3–6 months (when they switch from foetal to adult haemoglobin), causing growth faltering. There may be signs of extramedullary haemopoiesis, such as maxillary overgrowth and frontal bossing. These patients are dependent on transfusions.

- **Beta thalassaemia trait (minor):** Heterozygous form that is asymptomatic and results in a well-tolerated hypochromic, microcytic anaemia that is often picked up on routine bloods.

A key difference between beta thalassemia trait and iron deficiency anaemia is that ferritin is normal in beta thalassaemia trait and low in iron deficiency.

Sickle cell trait is the heterozygous (carrier) form of sickle cell anaemia in which patients have one abnormal allele of the beta gene. Haemoglobin Barts is the most severe form of alpha thalassemia in which all four alpha globin genes are defective causing intrauterine death because HbF cannot be produced. The other two types of alpha thalassaemia are HbH (3 defective genes), causing a microcytic hypochromic anaemia, splenomegaly and occasionally requiring transfusions; and alpha thalassaemia trait (1 or 2 defective genes), which is asymptomatic or causes a mild anaemia.

6. C

Congenital hypothyroidism occurs due to thyroid dysgenesis (absent or under-developed thyroid gland) or thyroid dyshormonogenesis (disruption of thyroid hormone production). It is usually identified soon after birth following the newborn heel prick test. If this is not performed, infants may present with excessive sleepiness, hypotonia, constipation, poor feeding and jaundice. Other associated signs include macroglossia and an umbilical hernia. If left untreated, infants will struggle to grow at a normal rate, and they may have a developmental delay. Severe cases, previously known as cretinism, are characterised by severe mental impairment and stunted growth. Thyroxine replacement therapy should be commenced within the first 1–2 weeks of life. Patients who are treated promptly can expect normal physical and mental development.

Constitutional growth delay is a delay in growth and the onset of puberty. It is the most common cause of short stature and pubertal delay in boys. Growth hormone deficiency should be suspected in children with a normal rate of growth in the first 6–12 months, followed by a drop in growth velocity. Cushing syndrome is rare in children and is usually iatrogenic (e.g. steroid therapy for asthma). Prader–Willi syndrome is an imprinting disorder that is associated with neonatal hypotonia, short stature, obesity and learning difficulties.

7. D

A baby undergoes immense physiological changes to their circulatory system immediately after birth as they go from having fluid-filled, non-functional lungs *in utero* to taking their first breath. *In utero*, the left atrial pressure is low as the lungs are full of fluid and very little blood returns to the left atrium. In addition, right atrial pressure is high as it receives the entire systemic venous return as well as blood from the placenta. The foramen ovale is a connection between the atria which allows blood to flow through the septum from the right atrium to the left atrium. This blood will then be pumped to the rest of the body.

When a baby takes its first breath, the fluid in the lungs is absorbed and the resistance to pulmonary blood flow falls rapidly and the volume of blood flowing through the lungs increases. This means that there is an increase in return from the lungs to the left atrium, so left atrial pressure increases. Meanwhile, disconnection of the placenta means that the volume of blood returning to the right atrium will fall. This change in pressure difference between the atria causes the foramen ovale to close. The ductus arteriosus, which remains open throughout intrauterine life to allow blood from the pulmonary circulation to enter the aorta, usually closes within a few hours or days but not immediately after birth.

8. B

If a child has collapsed and is not responding, it is essential to call for help, lie them on their back and maintain airway patency using manoeuvres such as head tilt and chin lift if necessary. Whilst maintaining an open airway, the rescuer should look, listen and feel for a breath for no longer than 10 seconds. If the child is breathing normally, they should be placed into the recovery position. If the child is not breathing normally (i.e. infrequent, noisy gasps may follow a cardiac arrest and should not be confused with normal breathing), 5 initial rescue breaths should be given. The child should then be re-assessed for signs of life for no longer than 10 seconds. This involves looking for movement, coughing or normal breathing and checking the pulse (carotid pulse in a child >1 year old and brachial pulse in an infant <1 year old). If signs of life are detected within 10 seconds, rescue breaths should be continued until the child starts to breathe effectively on their own. If there are no signs of life (including a pulse, <60 bpm) 15 chest compressions should be given immediately with 2 rescue breaths at a ratio of 15:2. Chest compressions should be given at a rate of 100–120 per minute and compressions should be sufficient to depress the sternum by at least one-third of the depth of the chest. In an infant, if possible, a thorax encircling grip with the thumbs on the middle of the sternum should be used. If this is not possible, the index and middle finger of the same hand can be used. In a child over the age of 1 year, the heel of one hand should be use. Chest compressions and rescue breaths should be continued until are child shows signs of life or further help arrives.

This child has already received 5 rescue breaths and is deemed to have no signs of life (since breathing is abnormal and pulse is <60 bpm). 15 chest compressions should, therefore, be administered.

9. A

Erythema nodosum is a panniculitis (inflammation of subcutaneous fat) which manifests as multiple, painful nodules on the shins. They are usually bright red when they first appear and will later fade leaving a purple bruise. It may be associated with a fever, muscle aches, malaise, and arthralgia. The causes of erythema nodosum can be broadly divided into three classes: drugs (e.g. combined oral contraceptive pill, NSAIDs, sulphonamides), systemic (e.g. sarcoidosis, pregnancy, inflammatory bowel disease), and infectious (e.g. streptococcal infection, tuberculosis, and mycoplasma infection).

Erythema multiforme is a hypersensitivity reaction that causes characteristic target lesions which starts on the hands and feet and spread along the limbs towards the trunk. 90% of cases occur due to infection, of which herpes simplex virus is the most common cause. Drugs such as NSAIDs, penicillins, and sulphonamides can also cause erythema multiforme. Erythema migrans is an expanding bull's eye-shaped erythematous rash seen at the site of a tick bite in patients with Lyme disease. Erythema marginatum is a feature of rheumatic fever and is a component of the JONES criteria along with joint involvement (migrating polyarthritis), myocarditis, subcutaneous nodules, and Sydenham chorea. Guttate psoriasis is a subtype of psoriasis that often follows a streptococcal throat infection or a viral upper respiratory tract infection. Lesions are small, raindrop-like, erythematous scaly patches on the trunk and upper limbs. The rash usually resolves within 3–4 months.

10. B

Obesity in children is diagnosed using BMI that is adjusted for age and gender. Children with a BMI at or above the 91st centile should have a tailored clinical intervention. Children with a BMI at or above the 98th centile should also be assessed for comorbidities, such as hypertension, dyslipidaemia, type 2 diabetes mellitus, sleep apnoea, joint problems, and exacerbation of chronic conditions. Children who are obese and have significant comorbidities should be referred to an appropriate specialist. To manage obesity in children, they should be encouraged to increase their level of physical activity to at least 60 minutes of moderate-intensity exercise per day. This should be accompanied by dietary changes to maintain an energy deficit. Children often respond well to behavioural interventions, such as setting realistic goals and rewards for reaching set goals. Drug treatment (e.g. orlistat) is generally not recommended for children under 12 years old and tends to be reserved for severe cases with comorbidities. Surgical intervention may be considered in children who have achieved or nearly achieved physiological maturity with severe obesity.

11. D

Hydatid torsion refers to twisting of the appendix testis (hydatid of Morgagni) — a vestigial remnant of the Mullerian duct located at the upper pole of the testis. This is the most common cause of an acute scrotum in children and tends to affect pre-pubertal boys. Although it is a benign condition, it presents similarly to testicular torsion with pain, erythema, and swelling, but the pain tends to be less acute than testicular torsion. These conditions need to be distinguished as testicular torsion requires urgent surgical exploration to reduce the risk of testicular necrosis. On clinical examination, the cremasteric reflex may be present in hydatid torsion and there may be a 'blue dot sign' (tender nodule with a blue discoloration at the upper pole).

Epididymitis presents similarly to torsion, but there is likely to be a history of dysuria or discharge from an ascending infection. The cremasteric reflex and Prehn's sign (relief when elevating the testicle) are also likely to be positive in epididymitis, but absent in torsion. However, it is clinically very challenging to distinguish between these three conditions and a Doppler ultrasound is the most appropriate 1st line investigation to assess testicular blood flow. Surgical exploration is mandatory in any acute scrotum unless torsion can be excluded with certainty. A hydrocele is an accumulation of serous fluid within the tunica vaginalis that presents as an asymptomatic and progressive scrotal swelling which transilluminates and surrounds the testicle. A varicocele is a dilation of the pampiniform venous plexus that may be asymptomatic or cause a dull ache. On examination, the lump may feel like a 'bag of worms' and does not transilluminate.

12. C

The management of asthma varies depending on the age of the patient. The main steps in the management of asthma, according to the British Thoracic Society, are outlined below:

>**STEP 1:** Inhaled short-acting beta agonist (e.g. salbutamol).
>**STEP 2:** If short-acting beta agonist is being used 3 or more times per week.

>- under 5 years old: start leukotriene receptor antagonist.
>- 5–12 years old: start paediatric-dose inhaled corticosteroid.

>**STEP 3:** Inhaled long-acting beta agonist (e.g. salmeterol) or leukotriene receptor antagonist.

STEP 4: Increase dose of inhaled corticosteroid or leukotriene receptor antagonist.

STEP 5: Refer for specialist care (e.g. oral steroids, omalizumab).

It is important to make sure that adherence and inhaler technique is assessed before stepping up the management. Non-pharmacological aspects of asthma management include providing a personalised asthma action plan detailing the steps that should be taken if the patient develops an asthma attack. Patients should also be advised about trigger avoidance and how to use a peak expiratory flow meter to monitor the severity of their asthma.

13. D

An epilepsy syndrome is defined by a combination of features, such as seizure characteristics, age of onset, EEG findings, genetic factors, and prognosis. Childhood absence epilepsy is characterised by absence seizures during which the child will stare into space and become unresponsive. An EEG will show fast generalised spike and wave patterns. It has a good prognosis and tends to go into remission in adolescence.

Infantile spasms (West syndrome) occurs in infants under 1 year of age. Patients will experience violent flexor spasms of the head, trunk, and limbs, followed by extension of the limbs which last a few seconds. EEG shows hypsarrhythmia. It has a poor prognosis and seizures are treated with vigabatrin and/or corticosteroids. Juvenile myoclonic epilepsy occurs in 12–18-year olds. Seizures can be myoclonic, tonic-clonic, or absence. Lennox–Gastaut syndrome occurs in 3–5-year olds and usually has multiple seizure types. Patients may also show signs of developmental arrest or regression and the EEG will show slow generalised spike and wave patterns. Childhood epilepsy with centrotemporal spikes (CECTS), previously known as childhood rolandic epilepsy, occurs in 4–10-year olds and is characterised by focal seizures often occurring at night with abnormal feelings in face and mouth. Most patients go into remission by adolescence. The EEG will show centrotemporal spikes.

14. E

Erythema infectiosum (also known as fifth disease or slapped cheek syndrome) is a viral exanthem caused by parvovirus B19. It typically presents with a 2–5 day prodromal phase, which is followed by a facial rash, resembling a 'slapped cheek' appearance. The rash may then spread to the trunk, back and limbs and eventually fades to produce a lace-like appearance. Management is conservative and includes adequate rest, encouraging fluid intake and simple analgesia. The child is no longer infectious once the rash develops and does not need to stay off school, but the school should be informed of the diagnosis to allow protective measures for at-risk groups.

Infectious mononucleosis (glandular fever) is caused by Epstein–Barr virus and should be suspected in children with fever, malaise, tonsillitis/pharyngitis, cervical lymphadenopathy, splenomegaly, and a non-specific rash. Measles, mumps, and rubella have become rare since the introduction of the MMR vaccine, but should also be considered as not all children have been vaccinated. Measles presents with a prodromal phase, followed by a fever, Koplik spots (white spots on the buccal mucosa), and a maculopapular rash that starts behind the ears and spreads down the body. Mumps presents with parotitis with non-specific symptoms, such as fever, headache, muscle ache, and appetite loss. Epididymo-orchitis is a potentially devastating complication that may occur one week later. Rubella presents with suboccipital lymphadenopathy, which is followed by a rash (starting on the face and spreading down the body), arthralgia, and non-specific symptoms.

15. E

Henoch–Schonlein purpura is a type of IgA vasculitis which typically presents with a purpuric rash over the extensor surfaces (particularly the buttocks and backs of the legs), arthralgia, and abdominal pain. It can also cause glomerulonephritis leading to proteinuria and haematuria. Although the cause is unknown, it is often preceded by an upper respiratory tract infection. Most cases will resolve spontaneously over several weeks. Joint pain can be managed using simple analgesia and oral prednisolone may be used in cases of severe scrotal oedema or abdominal pain. IV steroids may be considered in patients with nephrotic-range proteinuria. As the kidneys are affected, patients should be followed-up to check their blood pressure and renal function.

Meningococcal sepsis classically causes a non-blanching purpuric rash due to disseminated intravascular coagulation, however, patients would be acutely unwell with worrying vital signs. Idiopathic thrombocytopaenic purpura (ITP) is the most common cause of thrombocytopaenia in childhood and is caused by IgG-mediated destruction of platelets. It tends to occur within weeks of a viral infection and causes a purpuric rash, however, it would not cause the renal changes shown in this SBA, nor would the rash be limited to the buttocks. Thrombotic thrombocytopaenic purpura (TTP) is a disorder of blood clotting which is associated with five main features: microangiopathic haemolytic anaemia, thrombocytopaenia, reduced renal function, fever, and neurological signs. Haemophilia is an X-linked disorder of coagulation caused either by a lack of factor VIII (haemophilia A) or factor IX (haemophilia B). It tends to cause deeper bleeding into muscles and joints.

16. C

Premature thelarche is the development of breast tissue in females aged 6 months to 8 years in the absence of other signs of puberty, such as pubic hair and a growth spurt. In normal puberty, there will be an increase in the size of the breasts within 4–6 months of the first palpable breast disc appearing, but in premature thelarche, the breasts show little or no change in size and may become smaller. Since this is a non-progressive, benign condition without complications, parents can be reassured and followed up in 4–6 months to assess for signs of precocious puberty.

If there are signs of precocious puberty, further investigations are required, including measurements of gonadotrophins and sex steroids to differentiate between gonadotrophin-dependent and gonadotrophin-independent precocious puberty. An MRI head scan may be requested if an intracranial tumour (e.g. craniopharyngioma) is suspected as the cause of precocious puberty. Karyotyping is required to diagnose chromosomal abnormalities, such as Turner syndrome and Klinefelter syndrome, which are causes of delayed puberty. Gonadotrophin-releasing hormone analogues are used to treat confirmed precocious puberty due to the risk of early cessation of growth and reduced adult height.

17. D

Talipes equinovarus (clubfoot) is a fixed defect in which one or both feet point downwards and inwards, with the sole of the foot facing backwards. The affected side is often shorter and in 50% of cases, both feet are involved. It is usually idiopathic but can be genetic or occur secondary to neuromuscular conditions, such as spina bifida. The Ponseti method is the main treatment of talipes equinovarus, which involves manipulating the feet into the correct position and fixing them with a cast. This is repeated every week for 5–8 weeks followed by a minor operation to loosen the Achilles tendon. Talipes equinovarus needs to be distinguished from positional talipes in which the feet are in an abnormal position due to the cramped conditions *in utero* but can be corrected with passive manipulation.

Vertical talus is a rare birth defect in which there is a prominent calcaneus, midfoot dorsiflexion, and a convexly rounded sole (rocker-bottom feet). It is associated with neuromuscular or chromosomal abnormalities, such as spina bifida, cerebral palsy, Patau syndrome, and Edward syndrome. Pes planus (flat feet) occurs when the longitudinal arch in the foot has flattened or collapsed. This is often normal in young children but may be associated with cerebral palsy, spina bifida, and muscular dystrophy. Pes cavus is the opposite of pes planus, describing a high-arched claw foot and is associated with Charcot Marie Tooth disease and Friedreich's ataxia.

18. E

Pyloric stenosis is caused by idiopathic hypertrophy of the pyloric muscle resulting in gastric outlet obstruction. It usually presents between 2 and 8 weeks of age and is more common in boys. It presents with non-bilious vomiting, which increases in frequency and forcefulness, eventually becoming projectile. Vomiting occurs after every feed and the baby will remain hungry after vomiting. If it is not identified early, it can result in faltering growth. Physical examination may reveal an 'olive-shaped' mass in the right upper quadrant. A test feed may reveal peristaltic movements going from left to right across the abdomen. Regular vomiting in pyloric stenosis can lead to hypokalaemic, hypochloraemic metabolic alkalosis. Definitive treatment is with a Ramstedt pyloromyotomy which involves dividing the hypertrophic muscle.

Dystonic neck movements (torticollis) and arching of the back is describing Sandifer syndrome — a spasmodic condition associated with gastro-oesophageal reflux. Drawing up of the knees occurs in infantile colic and intussusception. A palpable 'sausage-shaped' mass is suggestive of intussusception. Palpation over the left iliac fossa that causes pain in the right iliac fossa is describing Rovsing sign — associated with appendicitis.

19. A

The initial treatment of eczema involves liberal use of emollients (including as soap substitutes), avoidance of triggers (e.g. allergens), and topical steroids for exacerbations. The emollients serve the purpose of acting as a barrier that prevents the skin from drying and becoming irritated. They should be applied frequently and over the entire body. Topical steroids, on the other hand, should be used short-term (usually less than 2 weeks) to bring an exacerbation under control. It should only be applied on affected areas. Topical steroids range in their strength as listed in the following table.

Strength	Drug
Mild	Hydrocortisone 1%
Moderate	Betamethasone valerate 0.025% Clobetasone butyrate 0.05%
Potent	Betamethasone valerate 0.1% Mometasone furoate 0.1%
Very potent	Clobetasol propionate 0.1%

If a certain steroid cream is ineffective at controlling the exacerbation, a stronger option is usually trialled. Topical calcineurin inhibitors (e.g. tacrolimus) may be considered as a 2nd line treatment option for eczema that is not controlled with steroids. In particularly severe cases with chronic lichenified skin, bandages may be applied to the affected areas. Antihistamines may be a useful adjunct in the treatment of eczema as it may help reduce itching and improve sleep.

20. C

Edwards syndrome is a genetic disorder caused by trisomy 18 and is the second most common trisomy (after Down syndrome). Most infants born with Edwards will die *in utero* or shortly after being born. Some physical malformations associated with Edwards syndrome include micrognathia, microcephaly with a prominent occiput, dysplastic ears, long fingers that overlap, rocker-bottom feet, and a shield chest. Children born with Edwards syndrome are prone to renal malformations, structural heart defects, omphalocele, and oesophageal atresia. For more information on eponymous syndromes, refer **Paediatrics: Paper 1, Answers Section, No. 28**.

Foetal alcohol syndrome is characterised by physical malformations, such as microcephaly, short nose, thin upper lip, epicanthal folds, and a smooth philtrum. Children may develop complications such as cerebral palsy, learning difficulties, poor growth, autism, and cardiac and renal malformations.

21. D

Epstein–Barr virus (EBV) causes infectious mononucleosis (glandular fever) which should be suspected in children with prodromal symptoms (e.g. malaise, chills, anorexia, and headache), prolonged fever, and sore throat. Examination may reveal tonsillar enlargement with a white exudate and palatal petechiae, splenomegaly, cervical lymphadenopathy, hepatomegaly, non-specific rash, and jaundice. In children older than 12 years of age and in the second week of illness, diagnosis can be made by finding more than 20% atypical lymphocytes on a blood film. In children younger than 12 years of age, EBV serology should be arranged after the child has been ill for at least 7 days. Management is symptomatic and consists of advising regular analgesia, bed rest, and adequate fluids. Exclusion from school is not necessary. Admission to hospital is required in children with suspected complications, such as dehydration or splenic rupture.

Scarlet fever is treated with penicillin V and patients should be excluded from school for 24 hours after commencing antibiotics. Whooping cough is treated with clarithromycin and patients should be excluded from school for 48 hours after commencing antibiotics. Amoxicillin (and ampicillin) should be avoided in children with suspected infectious mononucleosis as it causes a widespread maculopapular rash. Penicillin V and amoxicillin are used to treat group A streptococcal pharyngitis.

22. C

Choanal atresia is a rare congenital disorder in which the choanal openings (nasal passages) fail to form. Unilateral disease may be asymptomatic or present late with rhinorrhoea. Bilateral disease may present with neonatal respiratory distress as infants are obligate nose breathers. This may manifest as cyanosis or choking when the baby is feeding, as the oral route is obstructed and the infant struggles to coordinate feeding and breathing. Cyanosis is relieved on crying as it relieves the airway obstruction. Bilateral choanal atresia requires surgical correction.

Tetralogy of Fallot presents at 1–2 months of life with hypercyanotic spells during feeding or crying. An ejection systolic murmur may be heard at the left sternal edge. Transposition of the great arteries presents within the first few days of life with neonatal cyanosis without a murmur. Peritonsillar abscess (quinsy) is a complication of tonsillitis in which infection enters the space between the tonsillar capsule and superior pharyngeal constrictor muscle. It presents with dysphagia, voice changes, trismus, and excessive drooling. Laryngomalacia is a congenital abnormality of the cartilage in the larynx that results in partial collapse during breathing. It is the most common cause of stridor in infants.

23. C

It is important to carefully examine the genitalia during a neonatal examination as there are several abnormalities, such as hypospadias, undescended testes, and hydrocoeles, which benefit from early diagnosis and intervention. Hypospadias is a malformation in which the urethral meatus is not found in its usual location at the tip of the glans and is instead at a point along the ventral (bottom) surface of the penis. It arises from the failure of development of the ventral tissues of the penis or the scrotum. Surgical correction of hypospadias is not absolutely necessary, but it may be performed for functional or cosmetic reasons. It is, however, important to ensure that boys with hypospadias are not circumcised before a decision is made about surgically correcting the hypospadias, because the foreskin is sometimes used to repair the hypospadias.

Phimosis is a common condition in which the foreskin is non-retractile and cannot be pulled back over the glans. All boys are born with adhesions between their foreskin and glans which mean that their foreskin is initially non-retractile, however, as they grow older and develop erections, the adhesions will breakdown. Phimosis may result in an increased risk of infection. Paraphimosis is a condition in which a retracted foreskin cannot be reduced over the glans into its resting position. This is a urological emergency as it can reduce the blood supply to the glans. Labial adhesions are seen in baby girls and can be treated with topical oestrogens or steroids to help lyse the adhesions. Balanoposthitis is inflammation of the glans and foreskin.

24. A

Coeliac disease is caused by an immune reaction to the gliadin protein found within gluten. Intake of gluten-based foods like barley, wheat, and rye will lead to inflammation of the small intestines. It is initially investigated by testing for the presence of anti-tissue transglutaminase (anti-tTG) antibodies and anti-endomysial antibodies. A definitive diagnosis requires an endoscopy and duodenal biopsy. The characteristic histological feature is subtotal villous atrophy with crypt hyperplasia and an increase in intraepithelial lymphocytes. It often presents within the first 2 years of life when children are weaned onto gluten-containing solid foods. It can lead to persistent diarrhoea, bloating, features of iron deficiency anaemia, failure to thrive and wasting. It is treated by excluding gluten-containing food from the diet. This should result in resolution of the histological changes. Major risks of poor compliance with the diet include the development of enteropathy-associated T-cell lymphoma, iron, vitamin B12 and folate deficiency, hyposplenism, and osteoporosis.

Cows' milk protein allergy is an abnormal response of the body's immune system to a protein in cows' milk. These proteins can be transmitted through the breastmilk of a mother who consumes dairy products, or via direct consumption of dairy-based baby food. This typically presents earlier in life with a diverse range of symptoms including vomiting, eczematous rash, blood in the stool, and failure to thrive. Gastroenteritis is an infection of the gastrointestinal tract that is usually caused by a virus (e.g. rotavirus). It causes an acute episode of diarrhoea and vomiting and is typically self-limiting. Giardiasis is a protozoal disease that causes chronic diarrhoea, abdominal pain, and weight loss. Inflammatory bowel disease is a term that encompasses ulcerative colitis and Crohn's disease. They typically present with a variety of gastrointestinal symptoms (e.g. diarrhoea, bloody stools) in teenagers and young adults.

25. C

Status epilepticus is defined as either a single continuous seizure or repetitive seizures with no intervening recovery of consciousness lasting 5 or more minutes. This is an update of the old definition which defined status epilepticus as lasting more than 30 minutes. Status epilepticus is a neurological emergency and should be terminated as soon as possible. The algorithm for the treatment of status epilepticus is summarised by the following RevChart.

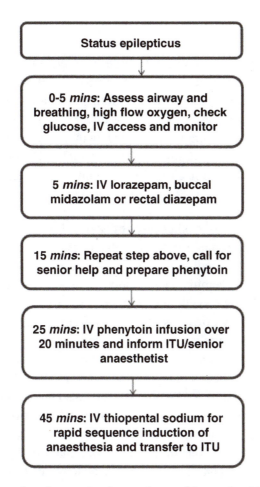

This child has already received one dose of buccal midazolam in the community, which has been unsuccessful. If still in the community, this could be repeated. However, as this child is in hospital and IV access has been established, the next most appropriate step is IV lorazepam. Once the seizure has been terminated, the underlying cause needs to be determined and treated. Febrile convulsions and epilepsy are the most common causes, but other differentials to consider include CNS infections, hyponatraemia, hypoglycaemia, cerebral vascular event, space occupying lesion, hypoxia, poisoning, and inborn errors of metabolism.

26. E

Duodenal atresia is a congenital absence or complete closure of the duodenum and is one of the most common causes of neonatal bowel obstruction. It usually presents with vomiting soon after birth which may be bilious dependent on the site of the affected segment of duodenum. Duodenal atresia is strongly associated with Down syndrome and an abdominal radiograph may reveal 'double bubble' sign (due to the presence of a distended stomach and duodenum with no gas distal to the affected segment). It requires prompt surgical correction.

Intestinal malrotation is another cause of neonatal small bowel obstruction resulting from abnormal rotation of the intestines during intrauterine development which predisposes to developing a volvulus. It may also present with bilious vomiting and abdominal distension, however, double bubble sign and Down syndrome are more strongly associated with duodenal atresia. Biliary atresia is abnormal development of the bile ducts that presents with jaundice, pale stools, dark urine and failure to gain weight. Gastroschisis is a congenital defect of the anterior abdominal wall adjacent to the umbilicus through which loops of bowel without a peritoneal covering will herniate. An omphalocele (also known as exomphalos) is a similar condition in which loops of bowel, with a covering peritoneal membrane, herniate through the umbilicus. Necrotising enterocolitis is inflammation and ischaemia of the bowel wall that usually occurs in premature neonates. It can cause vomiting, abdominal distension, bloody stools, respiratory distress, and peritonitis. Characteristic features on abdominal X-ray include distended loops of bowel, bowel wall oedema, and Rigler sign.

27. B

Head lice (pediculosis capitis) are small insects that infest the scalp and feed on human blood. They lay eggs which hatch and leave white egg cases (nits). If live head lice are found, wet combing should be recommended. This involves applying conditioner to the hair and then combing the hair with a detection comb. Wet combing should be done 5 times over

3 weeks. If no lice are identified at the final wet combing, the treatment is deemed successful. If wet combing is unsuccessful, physical insecticides (e.g. dimeticone 4%) which suffocates the lice or chemical insecticides (e.g. malathion 0.5%) which poisons the lice, can be used. These are applied twice, at least 7 days apart, and are followed by a detection combing. Children who are being treated for head lice can still attend school and there is no need to treat clothing or bedding that is in contact with lice. Permethrin 5% cream is used to treat scabies — a very itchy rash that is caused by a parasitic mite that burrows under the skin surface.

28. D

Cerebral palsy is a condition that is caused by a non-progressive lesion of the motor cortex that occurs around the time of birth. It is a spectrum of disease with patients being affected to different extents depending on the nature of the injury. It is primarily a motor condition leading to spasticity and difficulties with movement. Patients with cerebral palsy are at increased risk of epilepsy, gastro-oesophageal reflux, chronic constipation, behavioural and learning difficulties, and impairments of vision and hearing. Patients also tend to have trouble sleeping and produce excess saliva leading to drooling.

Cerebral palsy is incurable, however, there are treatment options available that can help achieve a better quality of life. Physiotherapy helps improve range of motion and strength. Speech and occupational therapy help patients improve their day-to-day functioning. Several medications may also be useful for symptomatic management such as baclofen for muscle stiffness, melatonin to help with sleep, laxatives for constipation, and anticholinergics to reduce drooling.

29. B

Gastroenteritis, typically presenting with diarrhoea and vomiting, is common in children and can lead to dehydration. Infants are at particular risk of dehydration leading to shock as they have a greater surface area to weight ratio, higher basal fluid requirements, and immature renal tubules. The most accurate measure of dehydration is the degree of weight loss: <5% weight loss suggests no clinically detectable dehydration, 5–10% weight loss suggests clinical dehydration, and >10% weight loss suggests clinical shock. If, as in this case, the degree of weight loss is unknown, clinical signs can be used as a guide. Signs of dehydration are listed in the following table.

No clinically detectable dehydration	Clinical dehydration	Clinical shock
Appears well	Appears to be unwell or deteriorating	Unwell or deteriorating
Alert and response	Irritable, lethargic	Drowsy, reduced level of consciousness
Normal urine output	Decreased urine output	Decreased urine output
Skin colour unchanged	Skin colour unchanged	Pale or mottled skin
Warm extremities	Warm extremities	Cold extremities
Eyes not sunken	Sunken eyes	Sunken eyes
Moist mucous membranes	Dry mucous membranes	Dry mucous membranes
Normal heart rate	Tachycardia	Tachycardia
Normal peripheral pulses	Normal peripheral pulses	Weak peripheral pulses
Normal capillary refill time	Normal capillary refill time	Prolonged refill time
Normal skin turgor	Reduced skin turgor	Reduced skin turgor
Normal blood pressure	Normal blood pressure	Hypotension

This child has signs of clinical dehydration, such as dry mucous membranes and reduced skin turgor, but a normal capillary refill, peripheral pulses, and blood pressure makes clinical shock unlikely. Hypernatraemic dehydration occurs rarely when water loss exceeds relative sodium loss, such as in extremely high fevers and hot, dry environments. This results in the movement of water from the intracellular compartment into the extracellular compartment which, if the brain is affected, can result in jittery movements, increased muscle tone, convulsions, and coma.

30. A

Pneumonia is an infection of the lung parenchyma that can have bacterial or viral origin. In children under 1 year, respiratory syncytial virus accounts for most cases. *Streptococcus pneumoniae* is the most common bacterial cause and other causative organisms include group A strepto-cocci, *Staphylococcus aureus* and *Haemophilus influenzae*. In older children, *Mycoplasma pneumoniae* should also be considered. Children with pneumonia typically present with a high fever and an increased respiratory rate (most sensitive marker). Other symptoms include lethargy, poor feeding, cough, vomiting, and chest pain. Examination may reveal cyanosis, increased work of breathing, coarse crackles, reduced breath sounds, and hypoxia. Children with signs of severe respiratory distress (e.g. oxygen saturation <92%, grunting, marked chest recession, cyanosis, respiratory rate over 60 breaths/min) should be urgently admitted to hospital.

All children with a clinical diagnosis of pneumonia should receive antibiotics as bacterial and viral pneumonia cannot be distinguished reliably. Amoxicillin is the 1st line oral antibiotic and macrolides (e.g. erythromycin) may be added if there is no response to initial treatment. For children who are not admitted to hospital, parents should be advised to seek medical advice if there are signs of respiratory distress, fluid intake is reduced to less than 75% of normal, the child becomes less responsive or the fever does not settle within 48 hours of commencing antibiotics.

Paediatrics: Paper 4

Questions

1. An 8-year-old boy presents to his GP with his mum who claims that, for the past few months, she has noticed that her son often needs things repeated to him and listens to the television on a very high volume. On examination, speech is normal, but there is gross hearing loss. Otoscopy reveals an air-fluid level behind the right tympanic membrane with loss of light reflex bilaterally. There are no signs of inflammation or discharge. How should this child be managed?

   A Prescribe a 7-day course of amoxicillin
   B Arrange hearing aids to be fitted
   C Arrange myringotomy and insertion of grommets
   D Active observation for 3 months and arrange hearing tests
   E Refer to an ENT specialist

2. A 5-year-old boy has had a limp for the last 3 weeks. He complains of some right-sided hip pain and, on examination, there is pain on abduction and internal rotation of the right hip joint and wasting of the gluteal muscles on the right. He has a past medical history of ADHD and he is in the 10th centile for height. What is the most likely diagnosis?

   A Developmental dysplasia of the hip
   B Osteomyelitis

    C Ewing tumour

    D Perthes disease

    E Slipped capital femoral epiphysis

3. A 4-year-old boy, who was playing in the waiting room of the outpatient clinic before an appointment, has suddenly developed an aggressive bout of coughing. He is crying and a wheeze is heard coming from his chest. What is the most appropriate first step in this patient's management?

    A Back blows

    B Abdominal thrusts

    C Encourage coughing

    D Call anaesthetist for intubation

    E Rigid bronchoscopy

4. A 9-year-old girl presents to A&E with acute abdominal pain and fever. She explains that the pain was initially central but has now moved to her right side. The pain is worse when she moves, and she has vomited 3 times. On examination, there is tenderness and guarding in the right iliac fossa. Appendicitis is suspected. Which investigation is most appropriate to confirm the diagnosis?

    A Full blood count and CRP

    B Urine dipstick test

    C Abdominal and pelvic CT scan

    D Abdominal ultrasound

    E Abdominal radiograph

5. A 12-year-old girl has wet herself at school several times over the past few years. She also has a 3-year history of lower back pain that worsens with activity. On examination, power is reduced in both legs and a sacral dimple is observed. What is the most likely diagnosis?

    A Spina bifida occulta

    B Meningocele

    C Myelomeningocele
    D Anencephaly
    E Encephalocele

6. A 12-year-old girl has been brought to A&E with severe breathlessness. On examination, she has a peak expiratory flow rate that is 30% of expected for her age. Her oxygen saturation is 85% on air and has been started on 15 L/min of oxygen via a non-rebreather mask. What is the most appropriate initial management option?

    A Nebulised salbutamol
    B Nebulised adrenaline
    C Nebulised tiotropium
    D Oral prednisolone
    E IV magnesium sulphate

7. A 1-week-old neonate is brought to the walk-in centre after developing a rash. On examination, he has several small white spots across his nose. He has been otherwise well and does not appear to be distressed by the rash. What is the most likely diagnosis?

    A Erythema toxicum
    B Naevus simplex
    C Naevus flammeus
    D Milia
    E Mongolian spots

8. A newborn baby has a head circumference that falls within the 99th centile. Which of the following is a potential cause?

    A Fragile X syndrome
    B Foetal alcohol syndrome
    C Patau syndrome
    D Craniosynostosis
    E Plagiocephaly

9. A 9-year-old boy is brought to A&E with a fever and a headache. On examination, he has a stiff neck and complains that the lights are making his headache worse. Blood cultures are taken, and a lumbar puncture has been arranged. His vital signs are shown below:

Temperature: 38.9°C
Blood pressure: 112/84 mm Hg
Heart rate: 102 bpm
Respiratory rate: 23 breaths/min
SaO$_2$: 99% on air

What is the next most important step in the management of this patient?

    A IV ceftriaxone
    B IM benzylpenicillin
    C IV fluid bolus
    D Supplementary oxygen
    E CT head scan

10. A 3-year-old boy has developed swollen eyelids and a swollen scrotum over the last 24 hours. He has recently recovered from an upper respiratory infection which was treated symptomatically by his GP. A urine dipstick and albumin: creatinine ratio is performed.

Urine dipstick: +++ protein – blood
Albumin: Creatinine ratio: 362 mg/mmol (<30)

What is the most likely diagnosis?

    A IgA nephropathy
    B Minimal change disease
    C Focal segmental glomerulosclerosis
    D Membranous glomerulonephritis
    E Renal amyloidosis

11. A 1-year-old boy presents to clinic with his father who claims that, since he has started walking, his shins and knees have been covered with bruises. He adds that his gums often bleed after he cleans his teeth. On examination, there is diffuse bilateral ecchymosis on the anterior aspect of the legs and knees. There is also a tender effusion in his right knee. His blood results are shown as follows:

Haemoglobin: 115 g/L (110–140)
Platelets: 212×10^9/L (150–400)
Activated partial thromboplastin time (APTT): 51 seconds (28–45)
Prothrombin time (PT): 12 seconds (10–14)
Fibrin degradation products: 2 mg/mL (<8)

What is the most likely diagnosis?

    A Von Willebrand disease
    B Haemophilia
    C Disseminated intravascular coagulation
    D Vitamin K deficiency
    E Idiopathic thrombocytopenic purpura

12. A 4-year-old boy presents to A&E with nausea, vomiting, and generalised abdominal pain. Examination reveals reduced skin turgor, sunken eyes, cold peripheries, and a capillary refill of 5 seconds. His plasma glucose is 12 mmol/l, VBG shows a pH of 7.2 and a urine dipstick shows ketones ++. A 10 mL/kg bolus of 0.9% saline has been administered. What is the next most appropriate step in the management of this child?

    A Start oral fluids
    B Start intravenous sodium bicarbonate
    C Start intravenous 0.9% sodium chloride with 40 mmol/L potassium chloride
    D Start intravenous 0.9% sodium chloride with 40 mmol/L potassium chloride and 5% dextrose
    E Start insulin infusion at 0.1 units/kg/hour

13. A 15-year-old boy presents with a 6-month history of loose bowel movements. He often notices blood mixed in with the stools. He has been feeling run down throughout this period and has struggled to maintain his appetite. He has lost 4 kg in weight. He has not changed his diet recently. A colonoscopy is requested which reveals terminal ileitis. What is the most likely diagnosis?

    A Crohn's disease
    B Ulcerative colitis
    C Irritable bowel syndrome
    D Meckel's diverticulitis
    E Coeliac disease

14. A young mother has brought her 1-week-old baby girl as her umbilical stump has become swollen. On examination, there is some redness and swelling around the umbilical stump. Her vital signs are shown as follows:

Temperature: 36.8°C
Blood pressure: 82/50 mm Hg
Heart rate: 152 bpm
Respiratory rate: 44 breaths/min

What is the most appropriate management option?

    A Topical fusidic acid
    B Topical hydrocortisone
    C Oral flucloxacillin
    D Oral benzylpenicillin
    E Blood cultures and IV antibiotics

15. A 6-year-old boy has developed a right-sided limp. On examination, there is symmetrical bowing of both legs below the knee and in-toeing. There is no tenderness, restriction of motion, or effusion. His vitamin D levels are within the normal range. What is the most likely diagnosis?

A Physiological genu varum
B Physiology genu valgum
C Osteogenesis imperfecta
D Blount's disease
E Rickets

16. A 9-month-old boy is brought to A&E by his father after having a seizure. His father explains that whilst playing on the sofa, he fell onto a carpeted flow sustaining a head injury. Immediately afterwards, his body became stiff and jerked a few times before regaining consciousness after about 15 seconds. What is the most likely diagnosis?

A Infantile spasms
B Epilepsy
C Febrile seizure
D Blue breath-holding spell
E Reflex anoxic seizure

17. A 2-year-old boy has developed red spots across his body. He has also had a fever and has lost his appetite. On examination, there are small, erythematous macules on his scalp, face, trunk and limbs, some of which have formed clear vesicles. Given the most likely diagnosis, how should this child be managed?

A Admit to hospital
B Prescribe oral aciclovir and advise that exclusion from school is not necessary
C Offer symptomatic treatment and advise exclusion from school until the lesions have crusted over
D Offer symptomatic treatment and advise that exclusion from school is not necessary
E Offer topical antibiotic and advise exclusion from school until the lesions have crusted over

18. Which type of hearing test is offered as part of the newborn hearing screening?

    A Tympanometry
    B Pure tone audiometry
    C Visual reinforcement audiometry
    D Automated otoacoustic emission test
    E Automated auditory brainstem response test

19. A 12-year-old girl with Turner syndrome is referred to cardiology after her GP incidentally noticed a systolic murmur at a routine follow-up appointment. She has not had any symptoms, but her GP noted her blood pressure as 145/98 mm Hg and an ambulatory blood pressure monitor has been arranged. What is the most likely cause of these signs?

    A Aortic regurgitation
    B Mitral regurgitation
    C Coarctation of the aorta
    D Aortic dissection
    E Hypertrophic obstructive cardiomyopathy

20. A 2-year-old boy presents to the GP with his mum because she is worried that his foreskin covers the tip of his penis. She denies any problems with urination but has observed some ballooning around the foreskin when he urinates. On examination, the foreskin is non-retractile and there are no signs of balanitis. How should this child be managed?

    A Topical corticosteroids
    B Oral flucloxacillin
    C Arrange circumcision
    D Reassure and advise gentle manual retraction of the foreskin
    E Reassure and advise against gentle manual retraction of the foreskin

21. A 2-year-old boy is brought to the paediatric A&E after developing a wheeze this morning. He has had a low-grade fever for the past 2 days with a runny nose and a cough. On examination, a wheeze is

audible, but the child is otherwise well. He has never had a wheeze before and has no past medical history. His vital signs are listed as follows:

Temperature: 38.0°C
Heart rate: 114 bpm
Respiratory rate: 30 breaths/min
Blood pressure: 98/62 mm Hg

What is the most likely diagnosis?

    A Asthma
    B Croup
    C Viral Wheeze
    D Multiple Trigger Wheeze
    E Bronchomalacia

22. A 10-month-old baby boy can reach out for objects and transfer them between his hands, but he cannot feed with a spoon or say any words. He has full control of his head but cannot sit unsupported. Which domain of development, if any, is delayed?

    A Gross motor
    B Vision and fine motor
    C Hearing, speech and language
    D Social, emotional and behavioural
    E Normal variant

23. A 15-year-old boy has developed acne across his face and shoulders which has failed to respond to topical treatments. The acne has had an impact on his confidence at school and he would like to step up his treatment. What is the most appropriate treatment to offer at this stage?

    A Benzoyl peroxide
    B Adapalene
    C Isotretinoin

   D Lymecycline
   E Metronidazole

24. A 2-year-old boy has developed frank haematuria and complains of abdominal discomfort. On examination, there is a large painless mass in the right flank. What is the most likely diagnosis?

   A Neuroblastoma
   B Alport syndrome
   C Wilms' tumour
   D Henoch–Schönlein purpura
   E Benign familial nephritis

25. A 10-day-old girl is brought to A&E after her skin turned yellow. She was born at 38 weeks' gestation, is being breastfed, and is otherwise fit and well. Her mum denies any fevers, weight loss, feeding difficulties, or changes in her stools or urine. Her serum bilirubin is 80 mmol/L (<350). What is the most appropriate management option?

   A Advise to continue breastfeeding and discharge
   B Advise to stop breastfeeding and discharge
   C Perform prolonged jaundice screen
   D Arrange phototherapy
   E Arrange exchange transfusion

26. A newborn baby boy has blue extremities, a pulse of 140 bpm, is actively moving, is crying loudly, and coughs on stimulation. What is his Apgar score?

   A 5
   B 6
   C 7
   D 8
   E 9

27. A 2-year-old boy is brought to the GP by his mother. He has been persistently itching his perianal region. This has been particularly troublesome at night and has been disrupting his sleep. What is the most appropriate management option?

    A Hygiene measures
    B Albendazole
    C Mebendazole
    D Doxycycline
    E Metronidazole

28. A 2-month-old boy has developed a thick, yellow, flaky rash on the top of his head. On examination, the rash is greasy and erythematous with some involvement of the eyebrows. The baby is otherwise well and does not appear to be disturbed by the rash. What is the most likely diagnosis?

    A Impetigo
    B Eczema herpeticum
    C Contact irritant dermatitis
    D Candida infection
    E Infantile seborrheic dermatitis

29. A 6-year-old girl has developed some abdominal pain that is localised around the umbilicus. She has also been going to the toilet more frequently and complains of a burning sensation when she urinates. On examination, her temperature is 38.4°C and there is some lower abdominal and loin tenderness on palpation. A urine dipstick is positive for leucocytes and nitrites. She has no significant past medical history. What is the most appropriate management option?

    A Refer urgently to a paediatric specialist for intravenous antibiotics and send urine sample for urgent microscopy and culture

B   Start oral cephalexin and arrange ultrasound during the acute infection

C   Start oral cephalexin

D   Start oral trimethoprim and arrange ultrasound during the acute infection

E   Start oral trimethoprim and arrange ultrasound during the acute infection and DMSA scan within 4–6 months

30. An 8-week old baby with Down syndrome presents with a history of bilious vomiting, constipation, and abdominal distension. On further questioning, he failed pass meconium within the first 48 hours of life. Which investigation is most likely to confirm the underlying diagnosis?

A   Abdominal ultrasound

B   Abdominal X-ray

C   Barium follow-through

D   Full thickness rectal biopsy

E   Oesophago-gastro-duodenoscopy

Answers

1. D

Otitis media with effusion (OME), also known as glue ear, is a collection of fluid within the middle ear space without signs of acute inflammation. It often occurs following an episode of acute otitis media. Hearing loss is usually the presenting symptom and some children may experience mild intermittent ear pain. If OME is bilateral, hearing loss may be severe and impact the child's development by causing a lack of concentration, social withdrawal, and speech or language abnormalities. Features of an effusion on otoscopy include loss of the light reflex, opacification of the drum, and an air-fluid level behind the drum. There should not be any signs of inflammation or discharge. Children with OME should be actively observed for 6–12 weeks as spontaneous resolution is common. During this period, they should have two hearing tests using pure tone audiometry and tympanometry. They should be regularly re-assessed for complication and changes in speech and language development. If features of OME persist, the child should be referred to an ENT specialist.

Myringotomy is the most common surgical option for OME. It involves making an incision in the tympanic membrane to drain the fluid, followed by insertion of grommets which stay in place for 6–12 moths to prevent recurrence. Myringotomy may be considered if symptoms have not resolved after 3 months. Antibiotics are not recommended for OME. Hearing aids may be offered to children with persistent OME as an alternative to surgical intervention.

2. D

Perthes disease is a condition in which the blood supply to the femoral head is temporarily disrupted resulting in avascular necrosis. For more information on distinguishing between Perthes disease and SCFE, please refer to **Paediatrics: Paper 3, Answers Section, No. 3**. In children under the age of 6 years, the prognosis of Perthes disease is very good and it can be managed with simple analgesia, bed rest, and physiotherapy. Severe cases may require surgery.

Developmental dysplasia of the hip (DDH) describes a spectrum of abnormalities of the neonatal hip joint, including dysplasia, subluxation, and dislocation. DDH is screened as part of the routine examination of the newborn and at the 6–8 week baby check. Osteomyelitis is an infection of the metaphysis of long bones, most commonly caused by *Staphylococcus aureus*. It presents with an extremely painful, immobile limb in a child who is unwell and pyrexial. The site of infection will be tender, erythematous, warm, and swollen. Ewing sarcoma is a malignant bone tumour that most commonly affects long bones. Presenting features depend on the size and location of the tumour, but bone pain is classically worst at night. There may be swelling or tenderness over the site and tumours may be incidentally discovered following a pathological fracture.

3. C

This child appears to have inhaled a foreign body that he was likely playing with in the waiting room. This should always be suspected in any case of abrupt-onset cough or wheeze in a child. The first and most obvious observation to make is whether the child is conscious or not. If the child is conscious, the following steps should be taken:

1. Encourage coughing
2. Back blows (×5)
3. Abdominal thrusts (×5)
4. Remove foreign body (rigid or flexible bronchoscopy)

In unconscious patients, CPR should be started immediately if breathing cannot be confirmed. Then, the airway should be secured immediately with endotracheal intubation. Then the foreign body should be removed using flexible or rigid bronchoscopy. In exceptional circumstances, surgery may be necessary. Untreated foreign body aspiration can lead to asphyxia, pneumonia, bronchiectasis, and atelectasis.

4. D

Appendicitis typically occurs in children and young adults and it classically presents with periumbilical pain that localises to the right iliac fossa, accompanied by fever, nausea, and vomiting. Young children may have vague and non-specific presentations. Full blood count and CRP are likely to reveal raised inflammatory markers, however, it is non-specific and does not confirm the diagnosis. The Alvarado score takes into account the leukocyte count, as well as the patient's signs and symptoms to determine the likelihood of acute appendicitis. A urine dipstick is useful to rule out a urinary tract infection, which is an important differential for abdominal pain. It may also be positive for leucocytes due to irritation of the bladder by the inflamed appendix. Abdominal radiography can only provide a diagnosis if an appendicolith (calcified deposit in the appendix) is visible but is useful for identifying free gas (from a perforation) or small bowel obstruction. Abdominal and pelvic CT is the most sensitive and specific investigation for appendicitis and will demonstrate a dilated appendix with a distended lumen and thickened walls. However, in children, ultrasound is the investigation of choice as it does not involve ionising radiation. In adolescent females of childbearing potential, it is also important to perform a pregnancy test to exclude ectopic pregnancy.

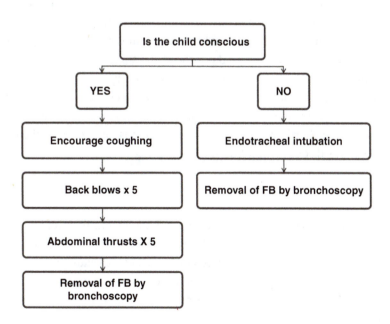

5. A

Spina bifida occulta is a neural tube defect that occurs due to failure of fusion of the vertebral arch. It is often an incidental finding on X-ray, but there may be an overlying skin lesion, such as a tuft of hair, lipoma, birth mark or dermal sinus. Tethered spinal cord syndrome is a complication of spina bifida occulta that describes fixation of the inelastic tissue of the caudal spine which causes abnormal movement of the spinal cord as the child grows. Disease progression is highly variable, but most develop an insidious onset of symptoms in childhood. Symptoms include lower back pain that worsens with activity, gait disturbance, scoliosis, high-arched feet, and neurological dysfunction (e.g. numbness or weakness, bladder and bowel dysfunction). Surgery is required to untether the spinal cord.

Meningocele and myelomeningocele are two other forms of spina bifida. Meningocele describes herniation of the meninges between the vertebrae forming a sac that contains cerebrospinal fluid. Neurology is normal since the sac does not contain neural tissue, but the sac is at risk of rupture, causing meningitis and hydrocephalus. Myelomeningocele is the most severe form of spina bifida and occurs when the spinal cord is able to protrude through an opening in an unfused portion of the spinal column. It is associated with severe neurological complications such as paresis, talipes, neuropathic bowel and bladder, and hydrocephalus. Anencephaly is the failure of development of most of the cranium and brain. Affected infants are usually stillborn or die shortly after birth. Encephalocele is herniation of the brain and meninges through a midline skull defect.

6. A

This patient is having a life-threatening asthma attack, features of which include peak expiratory flow rate (PEFR) less than 33% of expected, oxygen saturation less than 92%, altered consciousness, exhaustion, cyanosis, and silent chest. This patient requires urgent admission and should be given 15 L/min of oxygen via a non-rebreather mask as she is unable to maintain adequate oxygen saturation on air.

The 1st line treatment option for severe or life-threatening asthma is nebulised salbutamol. If ineffective, nebulised ipratropium bromide should be considered. A short course of oral prednisolone should be given to all patients with an exacerbation of asthma irrespective of severity as it helps reduce the inflammation within the airways. If these measures fail, an IV bolus of magnesium sulphate, salbutamol or aminophylline may be considered followed by an infusion of salbutamol and/or aminophylline. If all treatments are ineffective, intubation and ventilation will be necessary. After an exacerbation of asthma, it is important to review the management of the patient's asthma to check compliance with medication, inhaler technique and assess the need to step up their management.

7. D

Milia are tiny white cysts that contain keratin and sebum which appear as small white dots. It is a very common finding in newborns and resolves within a few weeks without treatment.

Erythema toxicum, although the name may suggest otherwise, is a common benign skin condition characterised by erythematous macules and papules which appear within the first few days of life and resolve spontaneously. Naevus simplex, also known as a salmon patch or stork bite, is a benign capillary malformation that is usually seen on the eyelids, glabella, or back of the neck. Most will disappear by the age of 1 year. Naevus flammeus, also known as a port wine stain, is a vascular malformation that does not regress. Patients require further investigation as it may be suggestive of a genetic syndrome such as Klippel–Trenaunay or Sturge–Weber syndrome. Mongolian spots are blue–grey birthmarks that are often seen in darker-skinned babies. It is often seen on the buttocks and back and are caused by a failure of migration of melanocytes through the dermis into the epidermis. Most Mongolian spots will disappear after a few years.

8. A

Macrocephaly is defined as a head circumference above the 98th centile and is associated with many genetic conditions, such as Fragile X syndrome, neurofibromatosis type 1, and tuberous sclerosis. Fragile X syndrome is an X-linked dominant disorder associated with characteristic physical malformations, such as a long, narrow face, large ears, and a prominent jaw and forehead. Other causes of macrocephaly include intraventricular haemorrhage, subdural haematomas, and congenital hydrocephalus, which may be caused by congenital infections (e.g. toxoplasmosis and syphilis).

Microcephaly is defined as a head circumference below the 2nd centile and causes include congenital infections (e.g. rubella and cytomegalovirus), foetal alcohol syndrome, and Patau syndrome. Craniosynostosis is a premature fusion of the cranial sutures which leads to distortion of the head shape. Plagiocephaly is unilateral occipital flattening, creating a parallelogram-shaped head. Brachycephaly is a similar condition in which there is bilateral occipital flattening. These two conditions are caused by infants spending an excessive amount of time lying on their back and usually resolve with time.

9. A

This patient is presenting with what is likely to be bacterial meningitis. Although a definitive diagnosis cannot be made without the results of the cerebrospinal fluid analysis, it is important to commence empirical antibiotics as soon as blood cultures have been taken as this disease can rapidly progress and is associated with serious morbidity and mortality if left untreated. As this patient is in an A&E setting, the best option would be IV ceftriaxone. In the community setting, IM benzylpenicillin is recommended and an ambulance should be called to take the patient to hospital. The patient is currently normotensive, not tachycardic and oxygenating well so IV fluids and supplementary oxygen would not be the priority in this case. Complications of bacterial meningitis include hearing loss, skin damage, and neurological problems. Patients should be reviewed by a paediatrician 4–6 weeks after discharge and a formal audiological assessment should be offered. It is important to distinguish between meningitis and meningococcal sepsis. Meningitis is, quite simply, inflammation of the meninges that can be caused by bacteria, viruses, fungi, and inflammatory conditions. Meningococcal sepsis, on the other hand, is an invasive bacteraemia that may or may not have a meningitis component.

10. B

Nephrotic syndrome is a condition in which the kidneys excrete excessive protein in the urine. It used to be defined as excretion of 3.5 g of protein/1.73 m^2 per day, however, since albumin: creatinine ratio (ACR) has superseded 24-hour urine collections, it is more often referred to as an ACR of more than 220 mg/mmol. Clinically, nephrotic syndrome is characterised by a triad of proteinuria, hypoalbuminaemia, and oedema. The most common cause of nephrotic syndrome in children is minimal change disease. It was given its name because renal biopsies show no obvious abnormalities on light microscopy, however, electron microscopy will show the loss of foot processes on epithelial cells. Most cases of minimal change disease will respond to a course of oral steroids (e.g. prednisolone for 4 weeks).

Focal segmental glomerulosclerosis is the most common cause of nephrotic syndrome in adults and is named based on the pattern of glomeruli affected — only a segment of each glomerulus is affected, and only a few specific glomeruli (i.e. focal) are affected. It is also thought to be due to an underlying defect of the epithelial cell foot processes, however, it is histological distinct as the affected areas become sclerosed giving a focal segmental appearance. Membranous glomerulonephritis is another cause of nephrotic syndrome, primarily in adults, which is caused by inflammation and damage of the glomerular basement membrane which is thought to be due to autoimmune attack. Renal amyloidosis results from the deposition of amyloid proteins in the kidneys, which can result in nephrotic syndrome. This is typically seen in patients with chronic inflammatory conditions or multiple myeloma and is unlikely in young children. IgA nephropathy is the most common cause of glomerulonephritis and tends to cause nephritic features (predominantly hypertension and haematuria) rather than nephrotic syndrome (predominantly proteinuria).

11. B

Haemophilia is the most common inherited coagulation disorder. There are two types, haemophilia A and B, both of which have an X-linked recessive inheritance pattern. Haemophilia A is caused by a factor VIII deficiency and is six times more common than haemophilia B, which is caused by a factor IX deficiency. The clinical features depend on the severity of the disease — mild disease is characterised by prolonged bleeding after minor trauma or surgery, whereas the hallmark of severe disease is recurrent spontaneous bleeds into muscles and joints, which can cause a crippling arthritis. Haemophilia often presents in the first year of life, as children are learning to walk, with haemarthrosis and bruising. Diagnosis and severity are determined by conducting a plasma factor VIII and IX assays. Classically, PT will be normal and APTT will be prolonged. It is treated with lifelong factor VIII and IX concentrates and desmopressin in mild haemophilia A.

Von Willebrand disease is an autosomal dominant deficiency of von Willebrand factor, which is involved with platelet-endothelial adhesion and protecting factor VIII from degradation. Blood tests will reveal a reduced factor VIII level, a prolonged APTT and normal PT. Although it may present similarly to haemophilia with bruising and prolonged bleeding, spontaneous soft tissue bleeding is rare. Disseminated intravascular coagulation (DIC) is widespread activation of coagulation and fibrinolysis that has a number of triggers, including sepsis, trauma, and malignancy. Blood tests will reveal a prolonged APTT and PT, thrombocytopenia, elevated fibrin degradation products, and schistocytes on the blood film. Vitamin K deficiency causes haemorrhagic disease of the newborn which presents with excessive bleeding from the umbilical stump, nose, and gums with a prolonged APTT and PT. Idiopathic thrombocytopenia purpura is IgG-mediated destruction of platelets that typically follows a viral infection and causes a purpuric rash with thrombocytopenia.

12. D

This child is presenting with diabetic ketoacidosis (DKA), a potentially life-threatening complication of type 1 diabetes mellitus (T1DM). DKA occurs due to a lack of insulin resulting in high blood sugar levels. This causes an osmotic diuresis resulting in polydipsia, polyuria, and dehydration. Insulin deficiency also promotes release of free fatty acids from adipose tissue, which are converted into ketone bodies in the liver. Ketone bodies are acidic and cause a metabolic acidosis. Kussmaul breathing is a deep breathing pattern which attempts to expel more carbon dioxide to compensate for the metabolic acidosis. Children with T1DM may also present with unexplained weight loss, abdominal pain, nausea and vomiting, and drowsiness. When a child presents with suspected DKA, it is important to measure their capillary glucose, capillary ketones (or urine ketones), and capillary or venous pH and bicarbonate. DKA is diagnosed when there is an acidosis (pH <7.3 or bicarbonate <18 mmol/L) and keto-naemia (blood β-hydroxybutyrate >3 mmol/L or ketonuria ++).

Children with DKA need to be admitted for treatment with early involvement of senior clinicians. Children who are alert, not vomiting and not clinically dehydrated, can be managed with oral fluids and subcutaneous insulin. All other children require intravenous fluids and intravenous inulin. If the child is in shock, a fluid bolus of 10 mL/kg of 0.9% sodium chloride should be administered. The total fluid requirement for the first 48 hours can be calculated by adding the estimated fluid deficit and the maintenance fluid requirement. When estimating the fluid deficit, a 5% fluid deficit is indicated by a pH >7.1 and 10% fluid deficit is indicated by a pH <7.1. Maintenance fluids are calculated using the reduced volume rules: 2 ml/kg/hour up to 10 kg, 1 ml/kg/hour for each kg from 10 to 40 kg and a fixed volume of 40 ml/hour if they weigh >40 kg. For example, a child weighing 15 kg should have $(2 \times 10) + (5 \times 1) = 25$ mL/hour. This is intentionally lower than standard fluid maintenance volumes to reduce the risk of cerebral oedema. The fluid deficit should be replaced evenly over 48 hours. 0.9% sodium chloride with 40 mmol/L potassium chloride is used for rehydration until the plasma glucose concentration is below 14 mmol/L, at which point 5% dextrose is added. The insulin infusion is started 1–2 hours after intravenous fluids are commenced.

13. A

Inflammatory bowel disease (IBD) is an umbrella term used to describe Crohn's disease (CD) and ulcerative colitis (UC). They both tend to present with rectal bleeding and loose stools in relatively young patients.

Although the underlying aetiology of the two diseases are incompletely understood, there are some key differences in the patterns of disease that helps distinguish them.

Domain	Ulcerative colitis	Crohn's disease
Presentation	Diffuse abdominal pain, rectal bleeding, and mucus	Right iliac fossa pain, failure to thrive between attacks, loose stools, and rectal bleeding
Examination findings	Clubbing, anterior uveitis, erythema nodosum, pyoderma gangrenosum, and signs of anaemia	
		Aphthous ulcers, fissures, and fistulae
Commonly affected areas	Rectum	Terminal ileum
Distribution	Rectum and colon	Any point from mouth to anus
Pattern of inflammation	Continuous lesions	Discontinuous (skip) lesions
Depth of inflammation	Confined to mucosa and submucosa	Transmural
Barium follow-through findings	Lead-pipe mucosa	Rose-thorn ulcers and cobblestone mucosa
Biopsy findings	Mucosal ulcers, goblet cell depletion, and crypt abscesses	Non-caseating granuloma
Management	Remission maintained with topical or oral aminosalicylates	Remission maintained with steroid-sparing agents (e.g. azathioprine)
Complications	Colonic adenocarcinoma and toxic megacolon	Abscesses, fistulae, adhesions, strictures, fissures, obstruction and perforation

The patient in this SBA has rectal bleeding and loose motions which could be present with both CD and UC. The colonoscopy findings showing terminal ileitis, however, confirms a diagnosis of CD.

Irritable bowel syndrome is a common condition which is generally used as a diagnosis of exclusion for inconsistent bowel movements which is not associated with red flag symptoms such as rectal bleeding or weight loss. Meckel's diverticulitis occurs when a Meckel's diverticulum becomes inflamed. It can mimic appendicitis by presenting with right iliac fossa pain, nausea and vomiting. Coeliac disease is caused by an immune response to the gliadin component of gluten. It typically presents in young children with failure to thrive and loose stools.

14. E

The umbilical cord is clamped and cut soon after birth, but a stump will remain until it falls off at about 1–2 weeks after birth. Infection of the umbilical cord is referred to as omphalitis. It presents with symptoms similar to cellulitis such as redness and swelling around the umbilical stump. There may also be pus coming from the umbilical cord as well as systemic features of infection (e.g. hypotension, tachycardia). There is a low threshold for intervention with umbilical cord infections as they can rapidly progress to sepsis. Even though this child has reassuring vital signs, it is important to escalate this case early and treat it aggressively. Blood cultures should be taken and IV antibiotics should be commenced. As the most commonly implicated organisms are *Staphylococcus aureus*, *Streptococcus sp.* and *Escherichia coli*, the preferred antibiotics are flucloxacillin and gentamicin. Keeping the umbilical stump of a neonate clean and dry will help reduce the risk of infection.

15. D

Genu varum is a bowlegs deformity in which there is an increased inter-condylar distance between the medial femoral condyles. Physiological genu varum is a common variant of normal stature in children under 2 years. If bowing persists beyond 3–4 years of age, it may suggest a pathological process such as Blount's disease or rickets. Blount's disease is caused by an abnormality of the medial aspect of the proximal tibial growth plate that causes slowly progressive bowing. There are two types of Blount's disease: infantile and adolescent. The infantile type affects children up to 3 years old, is usually bilateral, and most commonly affects the tibia. The adolescent type occurs in children over 10 years old, is usually unilateral, and involves both the tibia and femur.

Rickets refers to deficient mineralisation of the growth plates, most commonly caused by vitamin D or calcium deficiency. A small number of cases are caused by genetic mutations that cause defective vitamin D metabolism or vitamin D resistance. Rickets causes a number of skeletal abnormalities, including genu varum (in which there is medial angulation of both the femur and tibia), genu valgum (knock-knees), abnormalities of the metaphysis, short stature, frontal and parietal bossing, and rachitic rosary (expansion of the anterior rib ends). Osteogenesis imperfecta is a group of disorders that affect collagen metabolism and are characterised by osteoporosis, blue sclera, and hearing loss.

16. E

A reflex anoxic seizure is a type of breath-holding spell that typically occurs after a sudden shock (e.g. pain from a head injury). Patients are described as turning pale or grey, losing consciousness and becoming stiff. They then may have a generalised tonic–clonic seizure before regaining consciousness (usually within a minute). After the seizure, the child may appear drowsy or confused. They are caused by transient cessation of the heart due to excessive vagal activity. After a matter of seconds, the activity of the vagus nerve decreases and the heart will re-establish normal rhythm. Blue breath-holding spells are the most common type of breath-holding spell in which the child cries vigorously, holds their breath in expiration, turns blue and loses consciousness. This usually lasts for less than a minute at which point the child will regain consciousness and breathe normally. Patients should be reassured that neither type of breath-holding attack causes harm to the child. Nonetheless, it is important to definitively rule out a significant head injury by taking a detailed history and considering the mechanism of injury. A generalised tonic–clonic seizure following a head injury would require a CT head scan unless a diagnosis of reflex anoxic seizure is absolutely clear.

Febrile seizures are generalised tonic–clonic seizures which occur in febrile children. Infantile spasms (West syndrome) is an epilepsy syndrome characterised by violent attacks of flexor spasms of the head, trunk, and limbs followed by extension of the arms. They last a few seconds but are recurrent. Epilepsy is a tendency to recurrent, unprovoked seizures that can be diagnosed after a patient has two or more unprovoked seizures.

17. C

Chickenpox is a viral infection caused by varicella zoster virus. It typically has a prodromal flu-like phase, followed by a widespread rash consisting of small, erythematous macules on the scalp, face, trunk, and limbs, which progress to form intensely itchy clear vesicles and pustules. Vesicles will crust over within 5 days of the onset of the rash. The rash may be accompanied by fever, malaise, and feeding problems. Once the infection has subsided, varicella zoster virus persists in the sensory nerve root ganglia and can reactivate causing shingles. Chickenpox is usually self-limiting and complications (e.g. bacterial superinfection, meningitis, myocarditis, and pneumonia) are rare.

Children should be excluded from school or nursery until all the vesicles have crusted over. They should also avoid people who are immunocompromised, pregnant women and infants under 4 weeks old. Parents should be advised to ensure adequate fluid intake, keep their child's nails short and dress them appropriately (e.g. smooth, cotton fabrics). Symptomatic treatment should be considered, such as paracetamol, topical calamine lotion, and chlorphenamine. Oral aciclovir is only considered for children aged 14 years or older who present within 24 hours of rash onset and have severe chickenpox or are at risk of complications. If serious complications are suspected, the child should be admitted to hospital. Topical antibiotics are considered cases complicated by bacterial superinfection.

18. D

The newborn hearing test is carried out in the first 4–5 weeks of life using the automated otoacoustic emission test. This involves using an earpiece to play gentle clicking sounds and a detector picks up low-intensity sounds produced by the cochlea. If this suggests a hearing problem, the newborn is offered an automated auditory brainstem response test. Visual reinforcement audiometry is used in children aged 6 months to 2.5 years, pure tone audiometry is used to screen a child's hearing before starting school at 4–5 years of age and tympanometry is used to assess for otitis media with effusion (glue ear). The causes of hearing loss can be divided into sensorineural (lesion in the cochlea or auditory nerve) and conduction (abnormalities of the ear canal or middle ear).

19. C

Turner syndrome is a chromosomal disorder caused by the absence of a second X chromosome in females (45 X). The main features of Turner syndrome are short stature and a failure of development of secondary sexual characteristics. Patients with Turner syndrome will be amenorrhoeic, however they can develop secondary sexual characteristics and periods with the use of hormonal treatment. The lack of a full set of sex chromosomes also means that they are infertile although they may be able to conceive with assisted reproductive technology. Patients may present in infancy with lymphoedema of the hands and feet or webbing of the neck, but it may not be diagnosed until a failure of sexual development and growth is identified at a later age. Unlike many other chromosomal disorders, patients with Turner syndrome have normal intelligence, however, they have an increased risk of developing ADHD. Patients with Turner syndrome should undergo routine surveillance to check their cardiovascular health as it is associated with bicuspid aortic valve, aortic stenosis, and coarctation of the aorta. Coarctation of the aorta is a congenital narrowing of the aorta which is likely to be asymptomatic but may cause signs, such as hypertension and a systolic murmur heard loudest between the shoulder blades, which may be identified incidentally. Renal surveillance is also recommended as Turner syndrome is associated with structural renal anomalies (e.g. horseshoe kidney).

20. E

Phimosis refers to a condition in which the foreskin is too tight and cannot be retracted over the glans. At birth, baby boys will have adhesions between their foreskin and glans, however, by around the age of 2 years, the foreskin should start to separate naturally. Parents should be informed that phimosis at a young age is normal and they should be advised never to attempt manual retraction of the foreskin as it may be painful and damage the foreskin. Some parents may notice ballooning under the foreskin during urination, which occurs due to lysis of the preputial adhesions around the glans. Parents should be reassured that this has no functional consequence, does not imply obstruction, and does not require intervention. Phimosis can be problematic as it predisposes to inflammation of the glans and foreskin (balanoposthitis) due to colonisation with a mixture of organisms (*Candida albicans* being the most common). This presents with soreness, erythema, swelling, and discharge, and requires treatment with hygiene measures, topical hydrocortisone for non-specific dermatitis, topical imidazole for candidal balanitis, or oral flucloxacillin for bacterial balanitis. Another normal variant is the presence of bright red-orange urate crystals in the nappies of newborns. This is particularly common in breast-fed infants or infants receiving low volumes of fluids in the first days of life. They are often confused for blood and cause concern in new parents.

Topical steroids can soften the foreskin and are considered in pathological phimosis, such as in the case of balanoposthitis, problems with urination (e.g. dysuria, retention, and difficult urination), paraphimosis (foreskin gets stuck in a retracted position behind the glans), or urinary tract infections. Circumcision is recommended in rare cases, such as failure of steroid treatment to treat pathological phimosis, severe paraphimosis, and recurrent balanoposthitis.

21. C

A viral wheeze is a common cause of wheezing in pre-school children. As the airways of young children are small, inflammation due to a viral infection is more likely to lead to a significant narrowing that can cause breathing difficulties like wheezing. Patients with viral wheeze will only develop a wheeze whenever they have a viral upper respiratory tract infection, so it is important to check for symptoms such as cough, fever, runny nose, and viral exanthem. It can be treated with salbutamol through a spacer and follows the same escalation protocol as acute asthma (please refer to

Answers Section, No. 6 of this chapter for more information). Patients will be well in between viral infections.

Multiple trigger wheeze is a wheeze that can be triggered by several stimuli (e.g. cold air, dust, infections). A high proportion of patients with multiple trigger wheeze will go on to develop asthma. Patients tend to be classified as having asthma when recurrent wheezing is associated with symptoms in between viral infections (e.g. night-time cough) and there is evidence of an allergic responses to various allergens. The presence of other atopic conditions such as eczema, allergic rhinitis, and food allergy provide further support for a diagnosis of asthma. Bronchomalacia is a condition in which the cartilage supporting the bronchi is weak. It tends to present within the first few weeks of life with a wheeze and most patients will outgrow it by the age of 2 years. Croup is an upper respiratory tract infection that is usually caused by parainfluenza virus. It tends to present with a barking cough and stridor.

22. A

Please refer to the **Paediatrics: Paper 2, Answers Section, No. 27,** which lists key skills and their median and limit ages. At 10 months, a child would be expected to reach objects, transfer them between their hands, and sit unsupported. A child at this age may not yet have developed the ability to use a spoon or say any words.

23. D

Acne is a common condition seen in primary care. It most often affects teenagers who are going through puberty. The approaches to treating acne are based on targeting aspects of its pathogenesis. There are three main components that lead to the development of acne: increased sebum production (normal change seen during puberty), presence of *Cutibacterium acnes*, and blocked pores. Exfoliating face washes work by helping unblock pores, thereby reducing the build-up of sebum. Benzoyl peroxide is a topical agent that works by reducing sebum production, drying the skin, and having a bacteriostatic effect on *C. acnes*. It can be given in topical preparations combined with clindamycin or adapalene. Adapalene is a topical retinoid which has an exfoliative effect on the skin, thereby reducing blocked pores, and it has an anti-inflammatory effect on the sebaceous glands that are infected by *C. acnes*. Benzoyl peroxide (either on its own or in a combined formulation), adapalene, and azelaic acid are commonly used 1st line treatments for acne.

In patients with acne that is not responding to topical therapy, a course of oral antibiotics for a maximum of 3 months should be trialled. The two most commonly used antibiotics are lymecycline and doxycycline. If there is no improvement after 3 months, an alternative antibiotic should be trialled. If the patient has failed to respond to two courses of antibiotics or if there is evidence of scarring, the patient should be referred to dermatology to be considered for treatment with isotretinoin (often referred to by its brand name, Roaccutane). In female patients, the combined oral contraceptive may be used as an alternative to systemic antibiotics. Isotretinoin is a retinoid that is used to treat severe acne. It has several harmful side-effects (such as dry skin, depression, gastrointestinal bleeding, and muscle weakness) so is used sparingly.

The management of acne is summarised in the following RevChart.

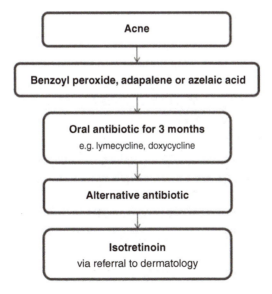

24. C

Wilms' tumour is a malignancy arising from embryonal renal tissue and is the most common renal tumour in childhood. 80% of cases occur in children under the age of five years and typically presents with a large abdominal mass and haematuria. Other features include abdominal pain, anorexia, and hypertension. It is treated with chemotherapy followed by nephrectomy, which carries an excellent prognosis.

Neuroblastoma is a tumour that arises from neural crest tissue in the adrenal medulla and sympathetic nervous system. Similar to Wilms' tumours, neuroblastoma often present with a large abdominal mass and features of metastatic spread, such as hepatomegaly, cutaneous lesions, proptosis, and skeletal pain/weakness. Alport syndrome is an X-linked recessive disorder of type IV collagen that causes a triad of nephritic syndrome, sensorineural deafness, and ocular disorders. Benign familial nephritis is also a genetic disorder of type IV collagen, but it is autosomal dominant and is usually diagnosed following the incidental finding of microscopic haematuria. Henoch–Schönlein purpura (HSP) is a small vessel vasculitis that causes a triad of palpable purpura, arthralgia, and abdominal pain. The vast majority of patients will also have renal involvement resulting in microscopic or macroscopic haematuria.

25. A

This patient has breast milk jaundice — a benign cause of jaundice of unknown aetiology. Breast milk jaundice typically presents in the first or second week of life with an unconjugated hyperbilirubinaemia in an otherwise healthy infant. All babies presenting with jaundice should have their bilirubin level measured urgently (within 6 hours) and this result is compared to a threshold table to determine management. Since this patient's bilirubin is below the treatment threshold, she is safe to be discharged and her mother can be advised to continue breastfeeding and reassured that the jaundice usually resolves by 4–5 weeks of age. In babies with jaundice lasting more than 14 days and with a serum bilirubin exceeding 100 mmol/L, a prolonged jaundice screen is required. This comprises a full blood count, conjugated bilirubin measurement, group and screen, Coombs' test, urine culture, and metabolic screening. This is to screen for other causes of jaundice, such as infection, congenital hypothyroidism, haemolytic disorders, and biliary atresia.

It is important to treat severe hyperbilirubinaemia to prevent kernicterus (encephalopathy from deposition of unconjugated bilirubin in the brain). Phototherapy uses light to convert unconjugated bilirubin into products that are more easily excretable in the stools and urine. During phototherapy, serum bilirubin should be measured every 4–6 hours, the eyes should be protected, and short breaks are encouraged. Phototherapy is stopped once serum bilirubin has fallen at least 50 mmol/L below the treatment threshold and serum bilirubin is measured 12–18 hours after stopping treatment to exclude rebound hyperbilirubinaemia. Exchange transfusion is considered if serum bilirubin is at potentially dangerous level and it involves removing blood from the baby and replacing it with donor blood.

26. E

The Apgar score is a neonatal assessment tool that looks at **A**ppearance, **P**ulse, **G**rimace, **A**ctivity, and **R**espiratory effort. It is measured at 1, 5, and 10 minutes after birth. The scoring system is outlined below.

Score	Pulse	Respiratory effort	Colour	Muscle tone	Reflex irritability
2	>100	Strong, crying	Pink	Active movement	Cries on stimulation/ sneezes, coughs
1	<100	Weak, irregular	Body pink, extremities blue	Limb flexion	Grimace
0	Absent	Nil	Blue all over	Flaccid	Nil

A score of 7 or above is considered normal. This infant has blue extremities (1), a pulse >100 bpm (2), is actively moving (2), is crying loudly (2), and coughs on stimulation (2). The Apgar score is therefore 9. This is likely to be describing a case of acrocyanosis — a benign condition that causes peripheral cyanosis immediately after birth in healthy infants and resolves within 48 hours.

27. C

Persistent anal itching in a young child is most likely due to threadworm (*aka* pinworm) infection. It is a common gastrointestinal infection caused by infection by the parasite *Enterobius vermicularis*. In children over 6 months old, the 1st line treatment option is a single dose of oral mebendazole. This dose may be repeated after 1 week if symptoms persist. As pinworm infections are extremely contagious, it is important to recommend hygiene measures such as regularly washing bedding and clothing at high heat and prophylactic treatment of household contacts.

28. E

Infantile seborrhoeic dermatitis (cradle cap) is a form of dermatitis that affects areas rich in sebaceous glands, such as the scalp and face. The rash is often described as being greasy with yellow scales. The rash is not itchy, and infants are otherwise well. It is self-limiting and usually resolves within several months. Treatment is conservative involving application of emollients or shampooing, followed by gentle removal of the scales. Hydrocortisone 1% may be used for extensive disease.

Impetigo is a superficial skin infection caused by *Staphylococcus aureus* which results in the formation of vesicles or pustules that later develop into honey-coloured crusted lesions. Eczema herpeticum is a complication of atopic eczema in which herpes simplex virus causes a disseminated skin infection. It presents with clusters of monomorphic blisters filled with a clear yellow fluid which eventually become crusted over. The lesions are itchy and painful. Contact irritant dermatitis often presents in infants as napkin dermatitis (nappy rash) due to prolonged exposure to urine or faeces, friction between the skin and the nappy or exposure to soaps and detergents. It appears as a well-demarcated erythematous rash that tends to spare the skin folds. *Candida* is a cause of napkin dermatitis which can be differentiated from contact irritant dermatitis as it may have satellite lesions and does not spare the skin folds.

29. C

If UTI is suspected in children under 3 months old, they should be referred urgently to a paediatric specialist for intravenous antibiotics, and a urine sample should be sent for urgent microscopy and culture. Children aged 3 months or older with acute pyelonephritis/upper UTI should receive a 7–10 day course of either oral cephalexin or oral co-amoxiclav. Children aged 3 months or older with cystitis/lower UTI should be given a 3-day course of oral trimethoprim or oral nitrofurantoin. Amoxicillin is a 2nd line option for cystitis/lower UTI. Any child with a high risk of serious illness should be referred urgently to secondary care. High risk features include mottled or blue skin, drowsiness, and respiratory distress. For more information on investigations used for recurrent or atypical UTI in children, please refer to **Paediatrics: Paper 2, Answers Section, No. 7**.

The management of UTI in paediatrics is summarised in the following RevChart.

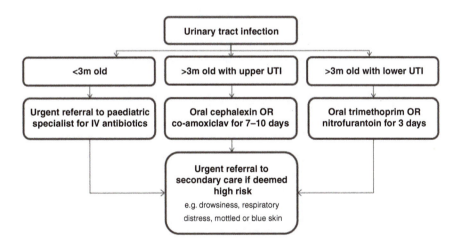

30. D

Hirschsprung disease is a bowel condition that is characterised by the absence of myenteric and submucosal plexus ganglion cells in the large bowel. The extent of bowel affected can vary. It tends to present in early life with failure to pass meconium within 48 hours, bilious vomiting, and abdominal distention. It is associated with Down syndrome and the presence of the RET proto-oncogene. It is diagnosed by demonstrating the absence of ganglion cells on a full thickness rectal biopsy. It is treated by performing an anorectal pull-through, which involves removing the affected portion of bowel. Down syndrome is also associated with duodenal atresia — a congenital anomaly in which part of the duodenum is blocked. As it is a complete blockage in the gastrointestinal tract, it would present much earlier.

Obstetrics and Gynaecology: Paper 1

Questions

1. A 37-year-old woman, who is 11 weeks' pregnant with twins, presents to the antenatal clinic with severe morning sickness. She is vomiting about 10 times per day, she has lost her appetite, and has lost about 5 kg of weight. She is feeling increasingly anxious about her current state. On examination, her mucous membranes are dry. What is the most appropriate management option?

    A Reassure that morning sickness will improve
    B Ondansetron
    C Metoclopramide
    D Cyclizine
    E Ginger and acupressure

2. A 24-year-old woman, who is 8 weeks' pregnant, presents with lower abdominal pain and vaginal bleeding. The pain began yesterday and has persisted overnight. On examination, the cervical os is open and blood can be visualised within the os. A transvaginal ultrasound scan reveals a gestational sac within the uterus with no foetal heartbeat. What is the most likely diagnosis?

    A Threatened miscarriage
    B Missed miscarriage

    C Inevitable miscarriage
    D Complete miscarriage
    E Septic miscarriage

3. A 42-year-old woman, who is 9 weeks' pregnant, is concerned about the risk of her child being born with Down syndrome and would like to know more about the screening test. Which factors are taken into account by the combined test for Down syndrome?

    A Nuchal translucency, PAPP-A, β-hCG
    B Nuchal translucency, unconjugated oestriol, β-hCG
    C PAPP-A, unconjugated oestriol, alpha-fetoprotein
    D Unconjugated oestriol, alpha-fetoprotein, inhibin A
    E Maternal age, nuchal translucency, inhibin A

4. A young couple are being managed by the fertility clinic as they have been unable to get pregnant after 3 years of regular unprotected sexual intercourse. Semen analysis reveals that the male partner has oligospermia. The mid-luteal progesterone of the female partner is within the normal range. A laparoscopy and dye test found patent fallopian tubes. Which of the following interventions is most appropriate in this scenario?

    A Clomiphene
    B Gonadotrophins
    C Intrauterine insemination
    D Intracytoplasmic sperm injection
    E Tubal microsurgery

5. A 32-year-old woman, who is 32 weeks pregnant, has been noted by the midwife to have a blood pressure of 154/98 mm Hg at her most recent antenatal visit. A urine dipstick is negative for protein, blood, and glucose. Her SFH is 33 cm. She has a past medical history of mild depression and asthma. What is the most appropriate management option for this patient?

    A No treatment needed
    B Labetalol
    C Nifedipine
    D Methyldopa
    E Hydralazine

6. A 23-year-old woman presents with a 3-year history of cyclical lower abdominal pain. The pain is severe and is often associated with heavy menstrual bleeding. She also experiences deep pain during sexual intercourse. Given the most likely diagnosis, what is the gold standard investigation?

    A Symptom diary for two cycles
    B Transvaginal ultrasound scan
    C Endocervical swab
    D Diagnostic laparoscopy
    E Magnetic resonance imaging

7. A 24-year-old woman, who is 14 weeks' pregnant, presents to her GP after her 4-year-old son developed chickenpox 3 days ago. She cannot remember whether she has had chickenpox before and is worried about the risk it poses to her baby. What is the most appropriate initial management plan?

    A No risk to the foetus at this gestation
    B Administer varicella zoster immunoglobulin
    C Urgent referral to foetal medicine specialist
    D Start oral aciclovir immediately
    E Check varicella zoster IgG

8. A 24-year-old woman attends a walk-in centre requesting emergency contraception. She had unprotected sexual intercourse 2 days ago. She would like to avoid invasive treatments. She has a past medical history of eczema and her body weight is 72 kg. What is the most appropriate treatment option?

    A Ulipristal acetate 30 mg
    B Levonorgestrel 1500 μg
    C Desogestrel 75 μg
    D Mifepristone 200 mg
    E Copper intrauterine device

9. A 32-year-old primiparous woman, who is 36 weeks' pregnant, has an ultrasound scan confirming that the baby is in breech position. The pregnancy has been uneventful thus far. What is the most appropriate management option?

    A Repeat scan in 2 weeks
    B Offer ECV immediately
    C Offer ECV at 37 weeks
    D Recommend elective caesarean section at 38 weeks
    E Recommend planned vaginal delivery at 39 weeks

10. A 32-year-old woman attends the fertility clinic with her partner. She has been unable to conceive for 2 years despite having regular unprotected sex. A blood hormone profile and a transvaginal ultrasound scan is requested. Which of the following hormone measurements indicates ovulation?

    A Early follicular phase FSH
    B Mid-luteal progesterone
    C Anti-Mullerian hormone
    D Prolactin
    E Oestradiol

11. A 26-year-old woman, who is 8 weeks' pregnant, presents with some concerns about fibroids in pregnancy. She was diagnosed with fibroids 2 years ago but opted for non-hormonal treatment with tranexamic acid as she was trying to get pregnant. Which of the following is a major complication of fibroids in pregnancy?

A Cystic degeneration
B Red degeneration
C Hyaline degeneration
D Placenta praevia
E Longitudinal lie

12. A 32-year-old woman presents to the GUM clinic complaining of painful blisters on her vagina. She claims she had unprotected sex last week after which she noticed some small, painful red lumps on her labia which transformed into blisters. She complains of some pain when urinating and burning around her vagina. She feels generally unwell and her temperature is 38.1°C. What is the most likely diagnosis?

A Genital warts
B Genital herpes
C Chlamydia
D Syphilis
E Gonorrhoea

13. A 34-year-old woman on the labour ward, who is 38 weeks' pregnant, has started having regular, painful contractions. She suddenly experiences a heavy gush of fresh red vaginal bleeding. On questioning, she has not experienced any pain aside from the contractions. The CTG shows late decelerations and foetal bradycardia. She had one previous delivery by emergency caesarean section. What is the most likely diagnosis?

A Placenta praevia
B Placenta accreta
C Placental abruption
D Vasa praevia
E Cord prolapse

14. A 64-year-old woman presents with a 2-week history of scanty vaginal bleeding. She went through menopause at the age of 53 years. A transvaginal ultrasound scan reveals an endometrial thickness of 12 mm. She is diagnosed with endometrial hyperplasia with no atypia following a hysteroscopy and biopsy. What is the most appropriate management option?

    A Combined oral contraceptive pill
    B Total hysterectomy
    C Endometrial ablation
    D Levonorgestrel intrauterine system
    E Repeat endometrial biopsy in 12 months

15. A 28-year-old woman, who is 32 weeks' pregnant, presents with a persistent itch in her hands and feet which is particularly bad at night. On examination, there are excoriations on her palms and soles but no obvious rash. What is the most likely diagnosis?

    A Normal feature of pregnancy
    B Irritant dermatitis
    C Hand, foot, and mouth disease
    D Scabies
    E Obstetric cholestasis

16. A 28-year-old woman presents to the gynaecology clinic with a 2-month history of lower abdominal pain and pain during sex. She has also noticed some intermenstrual bleeding. She had a copper intrauterine device inserted 1 year ago which she has been happy with thus far. Her observations are shown as follows:

Temperature: 37.2°C
Heart rate: 96 bpm
Respiratory rate: 14 breaths/min
Blood pressure: 94/62 mm Hg

What is the most appropriate management option?

   A Remove copper IUD immediately
   B Treat with antibiotics and review in 3 days
   C Treat with antibiotics and review in 1 week
   D Admit for IV antibiotics and arrange removal of copper IUD
   E Urgent transvaginal ultrasound scan

17. A 33-year-old woman attends her booking visit at 9 weeks' gestation. She has had one previous pregnancy which was complicated by gestational diabetes but was otherwise uneventful. What is the most appropriate management option given her past obstetric history?

   A Fasting blood glucose as soon as possible after booking visit
   B Fasting blood glucose at 24–28 weeks
   C Oral glucose tolerance test as soon as possible after booking visit
   D Oral glucose tolerance test at 24–28 weeks
   E Random blood glucose at booking visit

18. A 53-year-old woman presents with a 3-month history of urinary leakage. She describes the leakage of a small amount of urine whenever she laughs or coughs. This has caused her a great deal of anxiety leading to her restricting her fluid intake and going to the toilet to 'empty out' every hour. She has a past medical history of hypothyroidism and has had four children. What is the most appropriate initial management option?

   A Bladder retraining for 6 weeks
   B Pelvic floor muscle training for 3 months
   C Oxybutynin
   D Duloxetine
   E Autologous fascial slings

19. A preterm baby, born at 34 weeks' gestation, is jaundiced and has hydrocephalus. Further investigation finds sensorineural deafness, diffuse intracranial calcifications, and chorioretinitis. A congenital infection is suspected. The mother denies feeling unwell or experiencing any rashes during pregnancy. What is the most likely infectious agent?

    A Rubella virus
    B Cytomegalovirus
    C Listeria monocytogenes
    D Toxoplasmosis gondii
    E Varicella zoster virus

20. A 22-year-old woman, who is 13 weeks' pregnant, would like to terminate her pregnancy. She has found the pregnancy exceptionally stressful and would like to receive treatment that is most likely to rapidly and successfully terminate the pregnancy. What is the most appropriate management option?

    A Mifepristone and misoprostol
    B Methotrexate
    C Ulipristal acetate
    D Vacuum aspiration
    E Dilation and evacuation

21. A 31-year-old woman, who is 33 weeks' pregnant, presents to the GP with lower back and hip pain that worsens when walking and going upstairs. On examination, there is tenderness over the pubic symphysis. She has tried physiotherapy and some pelvic floor exercises but is still experiencing the pain and would like to check whether painkillers will be safe to take during pregnancy. How should the GP advise her?

    A It is safe to take ibuprofen and paracetamol together
    B It is safe to take ibuprofen
    C It is safe to take paracetamol
    D It is safe to take codeine
    E All painkillers should be avoided during pregnancy

22. A 62-year-old woman presents with a 5-month history of abdominal bloating and constipation. She has a past medical history of diabetes and used the combined oral contraceptive pill for several years to treat her painful periods. She went through the menopause at the age of 54 years. Her CA-125 is 64 U/mL (<35 U/mL). Which other investigation is necessary to calculate her risk malignancy index?

    A Transvaginal ultrasound scan
    B Biopsy
    C Fine needle aspiration
    D Blood hormone profile
    E Extent of weight loss

23. A 36-year-old woman, who is 12 weeks' pregnant with twins conceived by IVF, has presented to A&E with a swollen and erythematous left calf. She first noticed the swelling 6 hours ago and has not been feeling breathless. A compression duplex ultrasound scan confirms a DVT in her left popliteal vein. Which of the following is the most appropriate management option?

    A Treatment dose enoxaparin STAT
    B Treatment dose enoxaparin STAT followed by prophylactic dose enoxaparin for 3 months
    C Treatment dose enoxaparin STAT followed by prophylactic dose enoxaparin until 6 weeks' post-partum
    D Treatment dose enoxaparin for 3 months
    E Treatment dose enoxaparin until 6 weeks' post-partum

24. A 52-year-old woman is considering combined hormonal replacement therapy to treat the hot flushes and night sweats that she has been experiencing since undergoing menopause. She is concerned about the risks of hormone replacement therapy. What is the most appropriate information to give her?

    A There is an increased risk of colorectal cancer, weight gain, and heart disease

    B There is an increased risk of endometrial cancer, blood clots, and osteoporosis

    C There is an increased risk of endometrial cancer, weight gain, and dementia

    D There is an increased risk of breast cancer, blood clots, and gallbladder disease

    E There is an increased risk of breast cancer, colorectal cancer, and ovarian cancer

25. Which of the following is true regarding early decelerations on an intrapartum cardiotocograph?

    A Benign feature due to head compression

    B Indicates foetal asphyxia

    C Indicates cord compression

    D Associated with maternal pyrexia

    E Associated with placental insufficiency

26. A 26-year-old woman presents with a 3-month post-coital bleeding. She has one long-term partner and denies having sexual intercourse with anyone else. She is currently on the combined oral contraceptive pill and recently had her first cervical smear which was normal. Her abdomen is soft and non-tender, but speculum examination reveals a ring of erythema around the external cervical os. What is the most likely diagnosis?

    A Atrophic vaginitis

    B Cervical ectropion

    C Cervical polyp

    D Cervical cancer

    E Trauma

27. A 26-year-old primiparous woman, who is 40^{+3} weeks pregnant, is due to have an induction of labour tomorrow. She would like some more information about the process. What is the most common first step in the induction of labour?

    A Syntocinon infusion
    B Ergometrine infusion
    C Artificial rupture of membranes
    D Prostaglandin pessary
    E Prostaglandin gel

28. A 27-year-old woman attends an emergency GP appointment on a Monday morning. She is currently on the combined oral contraceptive pill and explained that she missed two pills over the weekend. She has taken this morning's pill and admits she had unprotected sex over the weekend. She is currently on week 1 of her pill packet. What is the most appropriate advice to give this patient?

    A Take the last missed pill and additional contraceptive measures are not necessary
    B Take both missed pills and use additional contraceptive measures for the next 7 days
    C Take the last missed pill, prescribe emergency contraception and advise that additional contraceptive measures are not necessary
    D Take the last missed pill, prescribe emergency contraception, and use additional contraceptive methods for the next 48 hours
    E Take the last missed pill, prescribe emergency contraception, and use additional contraceptive measures for the next 7 days

29. A 34-year-old woman, who just gave birth to a baby boy, has suffered a postpartum haemorrhage due to uterine atony. The estimated blood loss is 1500 mL. She was induced at 38 weeks' gestation due to worsening pre-eclampsia. She has just been administered IM syntocinon, however, the bleeding has continued. What is the next step in her management?

    A Administer IM ergometrine
    B Administer IM carboprost
    C B-Lynch suture
    D Balloon tamponade
    E Hysterectomy

30. A 29-year-old woman presents with a lump on her vagina. She explains that the lump has been there for a few months and was painless at first but has recently grown in size and become intensely painful. She tried soaking it in warm water, but this has not relieved the pain. On examination, there is an erythematous, fluctuant lump that is exquisitely tender on palpation. She has recently been feeling generally unwell and has developed a fever. What is the most appropriate management option for this patient?

   A Continue using warm compresses and use simple analgesia when needed
   B Prescribe antibiotics and arrange incision and drainage
   C Prescribe antibiotics and arrange marsupialisation
   D Prescribe antibiotics and arrange surgical excision of the Bartholin's gland
   E Prescribe antibiotics and arrange balloon catheter insertion

Answers

1. D

This patient has developed hyperemesis gravidarum — a severe form of morning sickness that is most pronounced in the first trimester. Hyperemesis gravidarum has three defining characteristics — more than 5% pre-pregnancy weight loss, dehydration, and electrolyte disturbance. If left untreated, hyperemesis gravidarum can lead to several complications including anaemia, malnutrition, venous thromboembolism, and depression.

The 1st line treatment option for hyperemesis gravidarum is an antihistamine such as cyclizine or promethazine. If these are ineffective, 2nd line options are ondansetron and metoclopramide. Steroids may be used in refractory cases. If patients wish to avoid pharmacological treatment, they may consider alternatives such as P6 acupressure on the wrist and ginger tablets. If patients are severely dehydrated, have ketonuria (3+) or have a severe electrolyte imbalance, admission may be required. In such severe cases, thiamine supplementation and thromboprophylaxis should be considered. It is also important to consider the effect of hyperemesis gravidarum on the psychological state of the patient and offer support where necessary.

2. C

A miscarriage is defined as spontaneous death of the foetus *in utero* before 24 weeks' gestation. There are several subtypes of miscarriage. An inevitable miscarriage is characterised by the presence of ongoing vaginal bleeding and abdominal pain with an open cervical os that may contain visible blood. This suggests that the patient is midway through the miscarriage and is likely to expel the pregnancy tissue without medical intervention.

A threatened miscarriage is when bleeding and pain occurs in early pregnancy, but the foetus remains viable with a visible gestational sac and foetal heartbeat on transvaginal ultrasound scan. A missed miscarriage is diagnosed by an absent foetal heartbeat on ultrasound or by lack of development of the pregnancy before pain and bleeding occur. On examination, the cervical os is closed. A complete miscarriage, as the name suggests, is when the patient has experienced abdominal pain and vaginal bleeding and fully expelled the pregnancy tissue. This means that, on examination, the cervical os will be closed and the uterus will be empty. A septic miscarriage is a surgical emergency when the products of conception become infected. In addition to abdominal pain and vaginal bleeding, the patient is likely to be showing features of sepsis.

3. A

The combined test for Down syndrome is offered to women between 10 and 14 weeks gestation. It takes into account nuchal translucency (measured at the dating scan), β-hCG (typically high in Down syndrome), and PAPP-A (typically low in Down syndrome). Based on these criteria and maternal age, a probability of having a child with Down syndrome is calculated. Any result with a higher probability than 1 in 150 is considered 'high chance' and patients will be invited to a follow-up clinic to discuss further investigations. The combined test will also generate a value for the probability of having a child with Edward or Patau syndrome. Late bookers who have missed the opportunity to have the combined test can be offered either the triple test (based on a combination of β-hCG, unconjugated oestriol, and alpha-fetoprotein) or the quadruple test (same as the triple test with the addition of inhibin A). These tests can be performed up to 20 weeks' gestation. Women with a high chance result should be offered chorionic villus sampling (available from 10 to 15 weeks) or amniocentesis (available from 15 to 20 weeks) for a definitive diagnosis. Cell-free foetal DNA (cffDNA) is a non-invasive technique that can be used to diagnose foetal genetic abnormalities and is available privately.

4. D

There are three main types of fertility treatment: medical, surgical, and assisted conception. Clomiphene is an ovulation-inducing agent that blocks oestrogen receptors in the hypothalamus and pituitary gland and increases the release of LH and FSH. Gonadotrophins or pulsatile gonadotrophin-releasing hormone are offered to women who have clomiphene-resistant anovulatory infertility. Mid-luteal progesterone is a marker of ovulation and, since the female partner has a normal measurement, the couple's subfertility is not due to anovulation. Tubal microsurgery is a surgical treatment of subfertility which involves tubal catheterisation or cannulation to resolve proximal tubal obstructions. The normal laparoscopy and dye test suggests that there is no tubal pathology.

Intracytoplasmic sperm injection (ICSI) involves injecting an individual sperm directly into an egg during *in vitro* fertilisation (IVF) to produce an embryo which is then transferred into the uterus. This method is suitable when the male partner has a low sperm count (oligospermia) or problems with maintaining an erection or ejaculation. Women under the age of 40 years can be offered three cycles of IVF treatment if they have failed to conceive after 2 years of regular unprotected sexual intercourse or if they have failed to conceive after 12 cycles of intrauterine insemination (IUI). IUI involves inserting sperm directly into the female partner's uterus. It is not usually offered in cases of oligospermia or poor sperm quality as it is unlikely to increase the chance of conception. Donor insemination involves using IUI with donor sperm and is considered in men with azoospermia (no sperm) on testicular biopsy or surgical extraction, if a partner has an infectious disease (e.g. HIV), if there is a high risk of transmitting a genetic disorder or same-sex couples. Oocyte donation is another method of assisted conception and involves IVF with donor eggs and is used in women with ovarian failure, bilateral oophorectomy or where there is a high risk of transmitting a genetic disorder.

5. C

Gestational hypertension is defined as the development of a blood pressure over 140/90 mm Hg with no proteinuria after 20 weeks' gestation in a woman with no previous history of hypertension. It is important to identify because, if left untreated, it can lead to pre-eclampsia, intrauterine growth restriction, and placental abruption. A blood pressure over 150/100 mm Hg requires treatment. The 1st line treatment option is labetalol, however, this patient has a past medical history of asthma which is a contraindication for labetalol. The next best option in this scenario would be oral nifedipine. Methyldopa is occasionally used if labetalol and nifedipine are contraindicated or poorly tolerated, however, the history of depression is a contraindication for methyldopa. Hydralazine may be used as a 2nd line intravenous treatment, however, it tends to cause a sudden and profound drop in blood pressure so patients may require pre-emptive administration of fluids. Patients with moderate gestational hypertension (150/100–159/109 mm Hg) should have their blood pressure measured at least twice weekly, and urine should be tested for protein at each antenatal visit. Patients with severe gestational hypertension (>160/110 mm Hg) should be admitted for treatment and monitoring until their blood pressure has come under control. Gestational hypertension typically resolves within 6 weeks after delivery.

6. D

Endometriosis is defined as the presence of endometrial tissue outside the uterine cavity. It is a common condition of unknown cause that affects 5–10% of women in their reproductive years. In endometriosis, the endometrial tissue is usually found within the fallopian tubes, but it can also be found within the ovaries (forming an endometrioma), peritoneum, and bladder. Endometriosis typically presents with cyclical pelvic pain that may be associated with heavy menstrual bleeding and deep dyspareunia. It can also cause dysuria and dyschezia (pain on defecation). Endometriosis can result in fibrosis and adhesion formation between pelvic organs and it is also associated with subfertility.

On bimanual examination, a mass might be felt (e.g. endometrioma) and the uterus may be fixed and retroverted due to the formation of adhesions. A transvaginal ultrasound scan may be useful to identify an endometrioma, however, it has a low sensitivity for endometriosis affecting other sites. A diagnostic laparoscopy is considered the gold standard investigation for endometriosis as it allows direct visualisation of the ectopic endometrial tissue. As this is an invasive procedure, most patients with suspected endometriosis will be treated using simple analgesia (e.g. NSAIDs), the combined oral contraceptive pill or progestogens to assess for an improvement in symptoms before subjecting them to a diagnostic laparoscopy. Endocervical swabs are used to identify bacteria, such as *Chlamydia trachomatis* and *Neisseria gonorrhoea*, which can cause pelvic inflammatory disease. A symptom diary for two cycles is recommended for patients with pre-menstrual syndrome.

7. E

Chickenpox (varicella zoster virus) in a non-immune pregnant woman can have catastrophic consequences. If it occurs before 20 weeks' gestation, it can cause congenital varicella syndrome which is characterised by cutaneous scarring, eye defects, limb hypoplasia, and neurological abnormalities. Pregnant women who have not had chickenpox before should be advised to avoid contact with anyone affected by chickenpox during the pregnancy. If a woman does happen to come into contact with chickenpox during pregnancy and they are unsure about their vaccination status, a test for varicella zoster IgG should be requested immediately. If the patient is non-immune, they should receive varicella zoster immunoglobulin (VZIG) provided that the exposure was within the preceding 10 days. It is also important to bear in mind that chickenpox is infectious from 48 hours prior to the onset of the rash, until the vesicles crust over (usually around 5 days after onset). If a pregnant woman develops chickenpox before 20 weeks' gestation, they should be treated with oral aciclovir and referred to a foetal medicine specialist 5 weeks after infection.

If maternal varicella infection occurs within 4 weeks of delivery, there is a significant risk of neonatal varicella. This is different from congenital varicella syndrome and it does not have any teratogenic effects, however, it can cause extensive cutaneous involvement, pneumonitis, and encephalitis. If birth occurs within 7 days of the onset of chickenpox in the mother, the neonate should receive VZIG and be monitored for signs of infection until 28 days after delivery. Neonatal varicella should be treated with aciclovir.

8. A

There are three main forms of emergency contraception: oral levonorgestrel (Levonelle), oral ulipristal acetate (ellaOne), and the copper intrauterine device. Levonorgestrel can only be used if unprotected sexual intercourse took place within the last 72 hours. Ulipristal acetate and the copper IUD can be inserted at any point within 5 days of expected ovulation. The copper IUD is considered the most successful option and it offers ongoing contraception, however, as this patient is keen to avoid invasive treatments, it would not be appropriate for her. This patient falls within the 72-hour window for levonorgestrel, however, in patients with a bodyweight over 70 kg or a body mass index greater than 26 kg/m², ulipristal acetate is preferred. Levonorgestrel could still be used in this patient but they would require a double dose (i.e. 3 mg). Both oral forms of emergency contraception work by inhibiting ovulation, thereby reducing the likelihood of fertilisation. The copper IUD has a spermicidal effect and causes sterile inflammation of the endometrial lining thereby preventing implantation.

Desogestrel is a progesterone-only pill that can be used for contraception but is not effective as emergency contraception. Mifepristone is a selective progesterone receptor modulator that is used in medical termination of pregnancy.

9. B

Breech delivery is a common complication of pregnancy that affects 3–5% of all pregnancies. Risk factors for breech presentation include uterine malformations, fibroids, placenta praevia, prematurity, and foetal anomalies. Although it is possible to achieve a safe vaginal breech delivery, it is associated with an increased risk of cord prolapse and perineal trauma. Breech presentations are usually identified when performing a pregnant abdomen examination, and it can be confirmed with an ultrasound scan. If it is detected before 36 weeks, no immediate intervention is necessary as it is probable that the foetus will move into a cephalic position by term. If still breech at 36 weeks, external cephalic version (ECV) should be offered immediately (i.e. at 36 weeks) for nulliparous women and at 37 weeks for multiparous women. ECV is a procedure that involves manually manoeuvring the baby into a cephalic position by applying pressure on the abdomen. It has a 50–60% success rate and is associated with a small risk of placental abruption and a risk of causing foetal distress resulting in emergency caesarean section. ECV is contraindicated if a caesarean section is required for another reason, the patient has had an antepartum haemorrhage within the last 7 days, the patient has an abnormal CTG, multiple pregnancy, or ruptured membranes.

If ECV is unsuccessful, both planned vaginal breech delivery and elective caesarean section are possible. Caesarean section is associated with a small reduction in perinatal mortality, however, it is associated with an increased risk of immediate complications for the mother (e.g. pain, wound infection, bladder injury). Caesarean section is also associated with a risk of placenta praevia and uterine rupture in future pregnancies. Deciding between planned caesarean section and vaginal breech delivery will be dependent on a number of factors including patient preference and past obstetric history (e.g. previous caesarean sections).

10. B

Patients who have failed to conceive after 2 years of unprotected sexual intercourse should be investigated further for an underlying cause. Several hormone tests are typically requested. After ovulation, the corpus luteum produces progesterone resulting in a high concentration of progesterone during the luteal phase (after ovulation). Therefore, the presence of a raised mid-luteal progesterone implies that ovulation has taken place and a progesterone-secreting corpus luteum has formed.

Menopause over the age of 40 years is a clinical diagnosis, however, in younger patients it is diagnosed by measuring the early follicular phase FSH. The loss of oestrogen production by the ovaries in menopause leads to a lack of negative feedback to the pituitary gland. This, in turn, results in a high FSH. Anti-Mullerian hormone is produced by granulosa cells within the ovary. It is important in regulating the development of follicles and is only present in the ovary until menopause. Therefore, it is a useful biomarker for ovarian reserve and helps predict the outcome of assisted reproduction. Prolactin is an anterior pituitary hormone that is important in the generation of milk within the breasts of lactating women. A high prolactin level is responsible for the contraceptive effect of breastfeeding. Pituitary tumours producing prolactin (prolactinomas) can mimic this effect, thereby causing difficulties conceiving. As such, prolactin may be measured when investigating a patient with subfertility. Oestradiol is the main female sex hormone which promotes thickening of the endometrium and, therefore, reaches its highest levels in the follicular phase (before ovulation) of the menstrual cycle.

11. B

Fibroids are benign smooth muscle tumours (also known as leiomyomas) that form within the wall of the uterus. In non-pregnant patients, it can cause heavy menstrual bleeding and subfertility. During pregnancy, fibroids can undergo a process called red degeneration. As the foetus and uterus grow, it begins to steal some of the blood supply that was previously supplying the fibroid. This results in ischaemia and necrosis. Red degeneration presents with severe abdominal pain typically during the mid-second trimester.

Hyaline degeneration is the asymptomatic softening and liquefaction of a fibroid. Cystic degeneration is asymptomatic central necrosis that leaves cystic spaces at the centre of the fibroid. Fibroids do not increase the risk of placenta praevia. Fibroids, especially if they are large, can distort the shape of the uterus and increase the risk of an abnormal (e.g. transverse) lie.

12. B

Genital herpes is a sexually transmitted infection (STI) that is caused by herpes simplex virus (HSV). Around 2–12 days following exposure, patients tend to develop painful, red lumps which turn into blisters within 24 hours. The blisters break, leaving shallow, painful ulcers that take 2–4 weeks to heal after the initial infection. This may be accompanied by dysuria and systemic symptoms, such as fever, malaise, and headaches. The virus enters the sensory nerves and lies dormant in the dorsal root ganglia. If reactivated, it tracks back along the nerve and causes a new herpetic eruption. Symptoms of recurrent outbreaks tend to be milder and shorter in duration and many patients have prodromal symptoms, such as localised genital pain or tingling before lesions appear.

Genital warts are benign, proliferative growths caused by the human papillomavirus (HPV) types 6 and 11 that can appear in the genital and perianal areas. Lesions may look like small, flesh-coloured bumps or have a cauliflower-like appearance. Chlamydia infection is the most common STI in the UK and is caused by the obligate intracellular bacterium *Chlamydia trachomatis*. It is usually asymptomatic. Gonorrhoea is an STI caused by *Neisseria gonorrhoeae* and may also be asymptomatic but can cause new vaginal discharge, dysuria, and dyspareunia. Both chlamydia and gonorrhoea can spread to the upper genital tract and cause pelvic inflammatory disease. Syphilis is an STI caused by *Treponema pallidum* and progresses through three stages. Primary syphilis is characterised by a painless ulcer (chancre) and regional lymphadenopathy. This may develop into secondary syphilis characterised by multisystem involvement with a generalised, maculopapular rash, generalised lymphadenopathy, and condylomata. Tertiary syphilis is a rare final stage that is subdivided into neurosyphilis, cardiovascular, and gummatous syphilis.

13. D

Vasa praevia is a condition in pregnancy where the foetal blood vessels run across the internal os of the cervix. They typically develop in this position due to velamentous insertion of the umbilical cord or the presence of an accessory placental lobe. The proximity of the vessels to the internal os means that, when the membranes rupture during labour, the blood vessels may bleed profusely. It typically presents with heavy, painless vaginal bleeding during labour. It is an obstetric emergency as the foetus is rapidly losing its blood supply which results in a pathological CTG trace. An immediate emergency caesarean section is necessary to prevent foetal exsanguination and death. Risk factors for vasa praevia include multiple pregnancy and *in vitro* fertilisation.

Placenta praevia also causes painless vaginal bleeding, however, the bleeding is mainly maternal and is unlikely to abruptly cause a pathological CTG trace. Furthermore, it is likely that a low-lying placenta would have been identified at the 20-week anomaly scan thereby allowing for closer surveillance of the condition. Placenta accreta is more likely to cause a postpartum haemorrhage as the placenta does not detach as easily after childbirth and some products of conception may be retained. Placental abruption typically causes sudden-onset severe lower abdominal pain with or without vaginal bleeding (depending on the position of the placenta). On examination, the uterus will feel large and tense. Depending on the extent of blood loss, the CTG may reveal foetal distress and the mother may go into shock. Cord prolapse would not cause heavy vaginal bleeding but is likely to cause CTG changes suggestive of foetal distress.

14. D

Although there are several benign causes of post-menopausal bleeding (most commonly atrophic vaginitis), it is important to investigate it further as a significant proportion of cases will be due to endometrial cancer. The most important initial investigation is a transvaginal ultrasound scan, which allows measurement of endometrial thickness. An endometrial thickness greater than 4 mm in a post-menopausal woman is considered abnormal and should be investigated further with an endometrial biopsy. The histological analysis will allow differentiation between endometrial hyperplasia with or without atypia, and endometrial cancer. Endometrial hyperplasia without atypia has a low risk of becoming malignant so does not require aggressive treatment. The 1st line treatment option would be to start continuous pro-gestogens (of which the levonorgestrel intrauterine system is considered the best option) as it promotes regression of the endometrium. The progesto-gens should be continued for a minimum of 6 months. Patients should also have endometrial surveillance (in the form of transvaginal ultrasound scans with biopsies) every 6 months. Reversible factors that contribute to endome-trial thickness (e.g. obesity, type 2 diabetes mellitus) should be addressed.

Endometrial hyperplasia with atypia has a much higher risk of progressing to endometrial cancer so requires more aggressive treatment. If preserva-tion of fertility is not necessary, a total hysterectomy is recommended. In younger patients who would like to preserve their fertility, progestogens and endometrial surveillance with biopsies every 3 months should be offered. Endometrial ablation is considered in patients with heavy men-strual bleeding who no longer need to preserve their fertility. The combined oral contraceptive pill should be avoided in this situation as it contains oestrogen which has a stimulatory effect on the endometrium.

15. E

Itching of the palms and soles which is worse at night with no rash is typical of obstetric cholestasis (also known as intrahepatic cholestasis of pregnancy). It is caused by an obstruction to the flow of bile through the biliary tree resulting in the accumulation of bile salts within the systemic circulation. The deposition of bile salts in the skin causes itching. The obstruction in the flow of bile will cause jaundice due to an increase in conjugated bilirubin levels in the blood, and it will also cause pale stools and dark urine. In severe cases, the lack of bile in the intestines leads to malabsorption of vitamin K (along with other fat-soluble vitamins) which can cause a derangement in coagulation. Obstetric cholestasis is associated with an increased risk of premature birth, stillbirth, and meconium passage, and therefore requires close monitoring. Aside from its characteristic clinical features, deranged liver function tests and raised bile acids support a diagnosis of obstetric cholestasis.

16. B

Pelvic inflammatory disease (PID) is an infection of the upper reproductive tract involving the uterus, fallopian tubes, and ovaries. Risk factors for PID include age (less than 25 years), multiple sexual partners, previous STI or PID, and the use of an intrauterine contraceptive device (IUD). PID can increase the risk of ectopic pregnancy, subfertility, and chronic pelvic pain, so it should be treated promptly. A course of antibiotics (ceftriaxone, doxycycline, and metronidazole) should be started immediately and the patient should be reviewed after 72 hours. If the symptoms have not improved in this time, removal of the IUD should be considered. As the patient is afebrile, IV treatment is not necessary at this stage. Patients should be advised against having sex until treatment is completed. A full STI screen, contact tracing and a discussion with the patient about contraception would also be recommended. A transvaginal ultrasound scan may be useful to rule out a tubo-ovarian abscess, which is an important differential, however, it would not be the most appropriate management option in this case.

17. C

Patients with a history of previous gestational diabetes mellitus (GDM) should be offered a 2-hour oral glucose tolerance test (OGTT) as soon as possible after the booking visit. If this result is not suggestive of GDM, a repeat test should be performed at 24–28 weeks. In patients with risk factors for GDM (obesity, previous macrosomic baby, family history of GDM or Asian, Afro-Caribbean or Middle-Eastern background), a 2-hour OGTT should be conducted at 24–28 weeks.

Patients with pre-existing type I or type II diabetes mellitus should have their HbA1c measured at the booking visit. Renal and retinal assessment should also be offered as increased insulin resistance during pregnancy is associated with an increased risk of poor blood glucose control and, hence, complications.

18. B

The patient is describing stress incontinence — a form of incontinence caused by an inability to keep the bladder outlet closed during slight increases in abdominal pressure. Patients typically describe leaking a small amount of urine whenever they do anything that increases their intra-abdominal pressure (e.g. laughing, coughing, lifting). Risk factors for stress incontinence include increasing age, multiparity, traumatic delivery, and obesity. The 1st line treatment of stress incontinence is 3 months of pelvic floor muscle training with a physiotherapist. Performing contractions on a daily basis will strengthen the muscles of the pelvic floor thereby improving the integrity of the bladder outlet.

Duloxetine is a serotonin-noradrenaline reuptake inhibitor (SNRI) that is usually used to treat depression. It can also be used as an adjunct to pelvic floor muscle training in patients with stress incontinence as it increases the activity of the urethral sphincter. If pelvic floor muscle training with or without duloxetine is ineffective or unacceptable, surgical approaches should be considered. Surgical procedures for stress incontinence include retropubic mid-urethral tape, urethral bulking agents, autologous fascial slings and Burch colposuspension.

19. D

Toxoplasmosis gondii is a parasite that can be transmitted from unwashed fruit and vegetables, raw or poorly cooked meat, unpasteurised goats' milk, and cat faeces. The vast majority of maternal infections are asymptomatic, but 40% will cross the placenta and cause congenital toxoplasmosis. Congenital toxoplasmosis only occurs with primary infection and transmission tends to occur in the 3rd trimester. Pregnancies are at increased risk of miscarriage, stillbirth, and preterm delivery. Most babies with congenital toxoplasmosis have no gross abnormalities but have delayed neurological and developmental sequelae (such as developmental delay, epilepsy, blindness, and deafness). 25% are still symptomatic at birth and may have a classic triad of intracranial calcifications, hydrocephalus, and chorioretinitis. Pregnant woman should be advised to wash fruit and vegetables properly and avoid handling cat litter, raw meat, and unpasteurised milk.

TORCH (**T**oxoplasmosis, **O**thers (e.g. varicella, listeria), **R**ubella, **C**ytomegalovirus, and **H**erpes simplex virus) is a mnemonic used to remember the congenital infections that can cause significant neonatal morbidity and mortality. All TORCH infections have similar non-specific findings, such as petechiae and purpura, hepatosplenomegaly, jaundice, small for gestational age, seizures, and haemolytic anaemia. Some distinguishing features of each infection are summarised in the following table.

Infection	Key points
Listeria	From soft cheese. **Features:** Spontaneous abortion, premature birth, pustular skin lesions, neonatal meningitis, and sepsis.
Varicella zoster virus	Congenital varicella syndrome occurs before 20 weeks. **Features:** Intrauterine growth restriction, premature birth, cutaneous scarring, cataracts, limb hypoplasia, and cortical atrophy.

(Continued)

(Continued)

Infection	Key points
Rubella virus	In unvaccinated mothers who present with rash, fever and lymphadenopathy. 90% of infections at 8–10 weeks' gestation will be transmitted to the foetus. Transmission is rare after 16 weeks' gestation. **Features:** Miscarriage, preterm birth, and foetal growth restriction. Classic triad of cataracts, cardiac abnormalities, and deafness at birth.
Cytomegalovirus	Only 10% symptomatic at birth; most have late complications. **Features:** Intrauterine growth restriction, chorioretinitis, periventricular calcifications, sensorineural deafness, and microcephaly.

20. D

Surgical termination of pregnancy is considered the most successful treatment option for gestations over 10 weeks. Vacuum aspiration is a procedure that involves gently dilating the cervix and using vacuum suction to evacuate the uterine cavity. The cervix may be ripened with misoprostol before the procedure. Vacuum aspiration can be performed up to 14 weeks' gestation.

If the gestation is greater than 14 weeks, a procedure called dilatation and evacuation is preferred. This procedure requires greater cervical dilatation to enable the removal of larger foetal parts. The contents of the uterus are evacuated using aspiration and forceps. An ultrasound scan will be performed to confirm complete evacuation. Medical terminations with mifepristone and misoprostol can be performed at any gestation but are most successful before 10 weeks' gestation. Ulipristal acetate is a form of emergency contraception that is ineffective once a pregnancy has been established. Methotrexate is the medical treatment of choice for ectopic pregnancy.

21. C

Pelvic girdle pain (also known as symphysis pubis dysfunction) is pain associated with excessive movement of the pubic symphysis due to laxity of the pelvic ligaments. It is initially treated using conservative measures, such as exercises to strengthen the surrounding muscles, warm baths, and support belts. Paracetamol is safe to use during pregnancy and is the simple analgesic of choice in pregnant women.

Ibuprofen is associated with an increased risk of miscarriage so should be avoided in pregnancy. It may be considered before 30 weeks' gestation in rare cases if the benefits are thought to outweigh the potential risks. After 30 weeks, it should be completely avoided as ibuprofen (and other NSAIDs) may cause premature closure of the ductus arteriosus, persistent pulmonary hypertension of the newborn, and oligohydramnios. Codeine is generally not recommended during pregnancy. If taken in the third trimester, it can cause neonatal withdrawal syndrome and neonatal respiratory distress. Other drugs that should be avoided during pregnancy due to their teratogenic effects include ACE inhibitors, angiotensin receptor blockers, methotrexate, warfarin, retinoids, and some antibiotics (e.g. trimethoprim, doxycycline, and tetracycline).

22. A

A change in bowel habit with abdominal bloating in a post-menopausal woman should always raise suspicion of ovarian cancer. Other symptoms include weight loss, vaginal bleeding, and loss of appetite. The risk malignancy index (RMI) is an algorithm that is used to assess the risk of a patient with an ovarian mass having ovarian cancer. This is based on three factors: Menopause status, CA-125 and findings on transvaginal ultrasound. CA-125 is a tumour marker for ovarian cancer, however, it may also be raised in several benign conditions including pregnancy, endometriosis, and alcoholic liver disease. The ultrasound findings that contribute towards the RMI are the presence of multiloculated cysts, solid areas, bilateral lesions, ascites, and intra-abdominal metastases. Patients with a high RMI should have a CT or MRI scan to characterise the extent of the disease and determine its operability. The treatment of ovarian cancer depends on its stage, however, the mainstay of treatment is a total abdominal hysterectomy with bilateral salpingo-oophorectomy with or without platinum-based chemotherapy.

Biopsy and fine needle aspiration are not performed for suspected ovarian cancer as disrupting the surface of the mass may increase the risk of metastasis. A blood hormone profile is unlikely to yield any helpful information in ovarian cancer. A notable exception, however, is that granulosa cell tumours may cause a high oestrogen level. Weight loss is a common feature of ovarian cancer, however, it is often difficult for patients to recall accurately and it does not contribute to the RMI.

23. E

The changes in clotting factors and the physical effects of a gravid uterus means that the risk of venous thromboembolism (VTE) is increased in pregnancy. Compounding risk factors include age (>35 years), obesity, multiple pregnancy, assisted reproductive technology, and a family history of VTE. Any pregnant woman with clinical features suggestive of VTE should be treated with treatment-dose low molecular weight heparin (e.g. enoxaparin) until the diagnosis is excluded. In patients with symptoms of DVT alone (like the patient in this SBA), a compression duplex ultrasound scan of the affected leg is the investigation of choice. In patients with symptoms of PE, a chest X-ray, ECG, VQ scan, and CT pulmonary angiogram may all be considered.

All patients with a confirmed VTE in pregnancy should be treated with treatment dose low molecular weight heparin for the remainder of the pregnancy and for at least 6 weeks postnatally and a minimum of 3 months in total. Women who are receiving this treatment should be advised that they should stop their injections when they go into labour. If they are having a planned delivery, the last dose should be taken at least 24 hours before. In cases of massive PE with cardiovascular compromise, IV unfractionated heparin is preferred.

24. D

Some of the benefits and risks of HRT are summarised in the following table.

Disease	Risk	Comments
Venous thromboembolism	Increased	2–4 fold increased risk with oral HRT. HRT patches or gels are not associated with this risk and patients with risk factors for venous thromboembolic disease may be offered these instead of oral therapy.
Breast cancer	Increased	Combined HRT is associated with an increased risk, whereas oestrogen-only HRT is associated with little or no risk. Oestrogen-only HRT does, however, increase the risk of endometrial cancer.
Cardiovascular disease	None	HRT does not increase the risk of cardiovascular disease when started before the age of 60 years. Oestrogen-only HRT is associated with no or reduced risk and combined HRT is associated with little or no increase in the risk.
Endometrial cancer	Increased	Oestrogen-only HRT is associated with an increased risk of endometrial cancer, but this is largely eliminated by continuous combined HRT.
Colorectal cancer	Decreased	HRT is protective against colorectal cancer and decreases the risk by about 1/3.
Gallbladder disease	Increased	Other factors may contribute to this, such as age, obesity, and silent disease.
Ovarian cancer	Unknown	There is conflicting results for whether HRT increases the risk of ovarian cancer and it is thought that if there is any risk, it is extremely small and disappears when HRT is stopped.
Osteoporosis	Decreased	HRT is effective in preserving bone mineral density, but lifelong HRT is required to be effective in preventing fractures.
Type 2 diabetes mellitus	None	HRT is unlikely to have an effect on blood glucose control.
Dementia	Unknown	NICE recommends that more research is required in this area.

25. A

Interpretation of a cardiotocograph can be done systematically using the mnemonic *DR C BRAVADO*:

- **D**efine **R**isk — why is the patient on a CTG monitor?
- **C**ontractions — up to 5 in 10 minutes
- **B**aseline **Ra**te — between 110 and 160 bpm
- **B**aseline **V**ariability — between 5 and 25 bpm
- **A**ccelerations — defined as a rise in FHR of at least 15 bpm lasting 15 seconds or more. Usually have two every 15 minutes usually occurring with contractions
- **D**ecelerations — defined as a reduction in FHR by at least 15 bpm lasting 15 seconds or more
- **O**verall impression

The main features of interest on a CTG are the foetal heart rate and the presence of different types of decelerations. The abnormalities and their potential causes are listed in the following table.

CTG finding	Causes
Baseline bradycardia	Cord prolapse, epidural/spinal anaesthesia, rapid foetal descent
Baseline tachycardia	Maternal pyrexia, hypoxia, prematurity
Reduced baseline variability	Hypoxia, prematurity
Early deceleration	Usually a benign feature caused by head compression during descent
Late deceleration	Foetal distress (e.g. asphyxia)
Variable deceleration	Sometimes due to cord compression

26. B

Cervical ectropion describes a physiological process in which glandular columnar epithelium (usually present on the endocervix) extends into the ectocervix (which usually consists of stratified squamous epithelium). This happens due to increased exposure to oestrogen (e.g. pregnancy, puberty, and combined oral contraceptive pill). Although most women are asymptomatic, it may cause an increase in vaginal discharge and post-coital bleeding because the columnar epithelium contains mucus-secreting glands and delicate blood vessels. Speculum examination may show a ring of erythema surrounding the external cervical os because of the increased vascularity.

The remaining options can all cause post-coital bleeding but are less likely given the patient's age and history. Atrophic vaginitis is thinning of the genital tissues that occurs most commonly after menopause due to the lack of oestrogen. Cervical polyps are benign growths on the surface of the cervical canal that are likely to be visible on speculum examination. Cervical cancer is unlikely as she recently received a normal cervical smear result. Trauma from intercourse is a potential differential, however, it is likely to cause some degree of dyspareunia and is a less common cause of post-coital bleeding in young women.

27. D

Induction of labour is a common occurrence on the labour ward. It is usually done in cases of post-term pregnancy and in the presence of any abnormalities (e.g. reduced foetal movements) in which the benefits of expedited delivery outweigh the risks. The first step in the induction of labour usually involves inserting a prostaglandin E_2 pessary. This is inserted for 24 hours and gradually releases prostaglandins which will ripen the cervix and stimulate uterine contractions. After 24 hours, if further cervical ripening is necessary, a prostaglandin gel can be inserted into the vagina on a 6-hourly basis. If these measures still haven't achieved sufficient cervical dilatation and uterine contractions, an amnihook can be used to perform an artificial rupture of membranes. Rupturing the membranes releases several cytokines which promotes further cervical ripening and strengthens uterine contractions. A syntocinon infusion may be considered if the strength of the contractions is inadequate. It can promote progress through labour by a phenomenon known as the Ferguson reflex — pressure on the cervix causes a release of oxytocin which stimulates uterine contractions thereby further increasing the pressure on the cervix. Syntocinon must be titrated judiciously with the frequency of contractions, as excessive use could cause uterine hyperstimulation which, in turn, can lead to foetal hypoxia. The usual sequence of induction of labour is summarised in the RevChart.

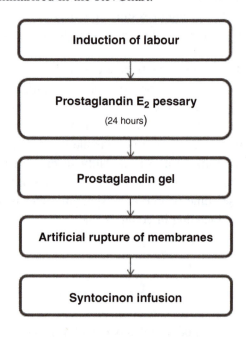

28. E

If a patient has missed only one combined oral contraceptive pill, they can be reassured that the contraceptive effect is still sufficient to prevent ovulation. They should, however, be advised to take the last missed pill (this may mean taking two pills on the same day). Emergency contraception and additional contraceptive measures are not necessary. If two or more pills have been missed, patients should be advised to only take one of the missed pills and discard any earlier missed pills. Additional contraceptive measures are recommended for the following 7 days. The need for emergency contraception varies depending on which week of the menstrual cycle the patient is in when they miss two or more pills:

- **1st week:** If the patient has had unprotected sexual intercourse in the preceding 7 days, emergency contraception is required.

- **2nd week:** No emergency contraception is required provided that the pills have been taken correctly for the preceding 7 days.
- **3rd week:** Omit the pill-free interval and start a new pack immediately after completion of the current pack.

Management of a missed progesterone-only pill (POP) is slightly different. Most modern POPs have a 12-hour window in which they need to be taken every day. Older POPs have a narrower 3-hour window. If the time window is exceeded, patients should be advised to take one missed pill only and the next pill should be taken at the usual time (this may mean taking two pills on the same day). Additional contraceptive measures should be recommended for the next 48 hours, as it takes time for the POP to sufficiently thicken cervical mucus. Emergency contraception is recommended if the patient has had unprotected sexual intercourse during this 48-hour period.

29. B

A postpartum haemorrhage (PPH) is defined as blood loss of more than 500 mL after childbirth. Blood loss in excess of 1000 mL is termed a major PPH. In the event of a major PPH, it is important to immediately call for help and alert the on-call consultant, anaesthetic team, haematologist, and transfusion lab. The patient should be laid flat, started on supplementary oxygen through a face mask, and 2 large bore cannulae should be inserted. Blood should be sent for a full blood count, clotting screen, group and save, and a crossmatch. A catheter can be inserted to help monitor urine output.

The first step in the pharmacological management of a major PPH is to administer IV or IM syntocinon. IM ergometrine or syntometrine are alternatives, however, they are contraindicated as this patient has suffered with a hypertensive disease during this pregnancy (pre-eclampsia) and they can cause a rise in blood pressure. If syntocinon is unsuccessful, IM carboprost (prostaglandin $F_{2\alpha}$ analogue) should be administered. Caution should be taken in patients with asthma as carboprost can precipitate bronchoconstriction. If carboprost is ineffective, a balloon should be inserted through the vagina and inflated to tamponade the uterus and reduce bleeding. The final step, if all else fails, involves surgical measures such as a B-Lynch suture or hysterectomy.

The step-wise management of PPH is summarised in the following RevChart.

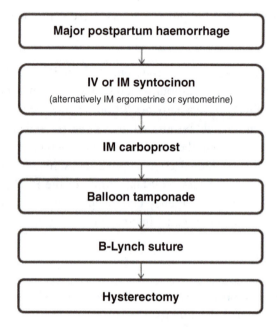

```
┌──────────────────────────────────────┐
│     Major postpartum haemorrhage       │
└──────────────────────────────────────┘
                    ↓
┌──────────────────────────────────────┐
│          IV or IM syntocinon           │
│ (alternatively IM ergometrine or syntometrine) │
└──────────────────────────────────────┘
                    ↓
┌──────────────────────────────────────┐
│             IM carboprost              │
└──────────────────────────────────────┘
                    ↓
┌──────────────────────────────────────┐
│           Balloon tamponade            │
└──────────────────────────────────────┘
                    ↓
┌──────────────────────────────────────┐
│             B-Lynch suture             │
└──────────────────────────────────────┘
                    ↓
┌──────────────────────────────────────┐
│              Hysterectomy              │
└──────────────────────────────────────┘
```

30. C

A Bartholin's cyst is a common benign lesion of the vulva caused by obstruction and consequent dilatation of the duct of the Bartholin's gland. Bartholin's cysts usually affect sexually active women between the ages of 20–30 years and typically presents with a painless swelling on the labia majora. Secondary infection results in a hot, erythematous tender lump called a Bartholin's abscess. Patients with a Bartholin's abscess may also complain of constitutional symptoms such as a fever.

Asymptomatic Bartholin's cysts can be managed conservatively with warm baths, compresses and simple analgesia, but persistent and symptomatic cysts may require surgical treatment. Balloon catheter insertion involves making an incision into the cyst to drain the fluid and insert a balloon catheter. The catheter is left in place for 4–6 weeks to allow epithelialisation of the tract after which the balloon is drained, and the catheter is removed. An alternative to balloon catheter insertion is marsupialisation in which the cyst or abscess is drained and a new mucocutaneous junction between the wall of the cyst and the skin of the labia is created to allow any fluid to drain without reforming a cyst. Broad-spectrum antibiotics may be used as an adjunct to these procedures. Surgical excision of the gland is considered a 2nd line treatment option and is reserved for patients with recurrent cysts or abscesses. 3rd line options include silver nitrate cauterisation, alcohol sclerotherapy, and laser ablation. Bartholin's abscesses should be treated with broad-spectrum antibiotics and referred for marsupialisation. Incision and drainage is often used to treat abscesses elsewhere in the body, however, marsupialisation is a better option for Bartholin's abscesses as it reduces the risk of reforming the cyst.

Obstetrics and Gynaecology:
Paper 2

Questions

1. A 34-year-old woman has just suffered a miscarriage at 8 weeks' gestation. She has had one previous miscarriage at 9 weeks' gestation and is yet to have a successful pregnancy. She has previously been able to get pregnant after 4–5 months of regular unprotected sexual intercourse, however, she feels disheartened after having a second miscarriage. She would like further investigation to identify the cause of her tendency to miscarry. Which of the following is the most appropriate next step in her management?

   A Screen for lupus anticoagulant antibodies
   B Transvaginal ultrasound scan
   C Cytogenetic analysis of patient and partner
   D Refer to fertility clinic
   E No further investigation needed

2. Which infectious diseases are routinely screened for as part of ante-natal screening in the UK?

   A Rubella, syphilis
   B Rubella, hepatitis B, HIV

    C Syphilis, hepatitis B, HIV

    D Hepatitis B, hepatitis C, group B *streptococcus*

    E Group B *streptococcus*, listeria, rubella

3. A 17-year-old girl presents to her GP with a 6-month history of mood swings and difficulty sleeping. The symptoms mainly occur in the week before her period begins during which she feels tearful and irritable. She says that she is generally able to keep up with her day-to-day activities but has found it more difficult to concentrate at school because of her symptoms. She describes her periods as being heavy but not painful. She would like treatment to lessen the symptoms in the build up to her exams. What is the most appropriate management option?

    A Combined oral contraceptive pill

    B Fluoxetine

    C Contraceptive implant

    D GnRH analogue

    E Sleep hygiene advice

4. A 26-year-old woman, who gave birth to a baby girl 6 weeks ago, has presented with a painful right breast. On examination, the right breast is red, swollen and tender, and the nipple is fissured. She has felt constantly tired since giving birth. What is the most appropriate management option?

    A Encourage continued breastfeeding only

    B Oral flucloxacillin and stop breastfeeding

    C Oral flucloxacillin and continue breastfeeding

    D Topical miconazole and stop breastfeeding

    E Incision and drainage

5. A 65-year-old woman has been diagnosed with an ovarian tumour after presenting with post-menopausal bleeding and bloating. She is informed that that the tumour is a functioning tumour that produces oestrogen, so she is at an increased risk of endometrial carcinoma.

Histology reports the presence of Call–Exner bodies. What is the most likely underlying diagnosis?

    A Granulosa cell tumour
    B Sertoli–Leydig cell tumour
    C Dysgerminoma
    D Fibroma
    E Krukenberg tumour

6. A 33-year-old woman, who is 24 weeks pregnant is referred for blood glucose testing after glycosuria was detected on a urine dipstick. The results of the blood glucose tests are shown in the following:

Fasting blood glucose: 7.3 mmol/L
2-hour OGTT: 10.7 mmol/L

What is the most appropriate management option?

    A Lifestyle modification
    B Metformin
    C Insulin
    D Glibenclamide
    E Acarbose

7. A 29-year-old woman has failed to get pregnant despite having regular unprotected sex for 2 years. She is otherwise asymptomatic with regular menstrual cycles of 28 days and has no significant past medical history. Which panel of investigations should be ordered first?

    A Semen analysis, screen both partners for chlamydia and measure serum progesterone, gonadotrophins, thyroid function, and prolactin
    B Semen analysis, screen both partners for chlamydia and measure mid-luteal phase progesterone
    C Semen analysis and advise basal body temperature charts

    D Screen both partners for chlamydia and measure serum progesterone, gonadotrophins, thyroid function, and prolactin

    E Screen both partners for chlamydia, advise basal body temperature charts, and measure mid-luteal phase progesterone

8. A 31-year-old woman presents for an antenatal visit at 34 weeks' gestation. She mentions that her bump has grown more than she was expecting in the past few weeks. An ultrasound scan reveals an amniotic fluid index of 26 cm. Which of the following is a potential cause of this condition?

    A Foetal duodenal atresia
    B Pre-eclampsia
    C Foetal renal agenesis
    D Post-dates pregnancy
    E Intrauterine growth restriction

9. A 36-year-old woman, with a history of migraine with aura, attends her GP practice to discuss her contraceptive options. She is aware that given her migraines, she will be unable to receive the combined oral contraceptive pill and would like to receive the progesterone-only pill. What is the mechanism of action of the progesterone-only pill?

    A Prevents ovulation
    B Prevents implantation
    C Thins the endometrium
    D Thickens cervical mucus
    E Kills sperm

10. A 21-year-old woman goes into labour at 35 weeks' gestation. On examination, the cervix is 6 cm dilated, the foetal head is 3/5 engaged, and the umbilical cord is palpated below the presenting part. A CTG reveals a foetal baseline heart rate of 96 bpm. How should this patient be managed?

A Elevate the cord, adopt the knee-chest position and arrange immediate caesarean section
B Elevate the presenting part, adopt the knee-to-chest position, and arrange immediate caesarean section
C Adopt McRoberts manoeuvre and apply suprapubic pressure
D Immediate instrumental delivery
E Artificial rupture of membranes

11. A 26-year-old woman presents to her GP with a 9-month history of irregular periods. Her cycles can vary in length from 28–60 days. She suffered from heavy and irregular periods as a teenager but managed to gain control of her periods using the combined oral contraceptive pill. She has not taken the pill for the last 14 months as she has been trying to get pregnant. She has a family history of type 2 diabetes mellitus and a recent fasting blood glucose test revealed impaired fasting glucose. Which investigation is most likely to reveal the underlying diagnosis?

A Thyroid function tests
B Transvaginal ultrasound scan
C Urine pregnancy test
D 9 am cortisol
E Mid-luteal progesterone

12. A 22-year-old woman, who is 9 weeks' pregnant, attends her booking visit. She is anxious about the prospect of labour and is interested in finding out more about having a planned caesarean section. Which of the following is an indication for offering a planned caesarean section?

A Multiple pregnancy in which the first twin is cephalic
B HIV-positive women who are receiving anti-retroviral therapy with a viral load of 40 copies/ml
C Women who have a classical caesarean section scar
D Women with primary genital herpes simplex virus infection occurring in the 2nd trimester
E Women who have a chronic hepatitis C infection

13. A 62-year-old woman with post-menopausal bleeding is found to have increased endometrial thickness on transvaginal ultrasound. A hysteroscopy and biopsy is performed and endometrial hyperplasia is diagnosed. Which of the following is not a risk factor for endometrial hyperplasia?

    A Nulliparity
    B Early menarche
    C Combined oral contraception
    D Tamoxifen
    E Obesity

14. A 31-year-old woman, who is 34 weeks' pregnant, presents with an itch that is worse at night. A diagnosis of obstetric cholestasis is suspected. How should this patient be managed?

    A Offer topical emollients and cholestyramine
    B Offer topical emollients and antihistamines
    C Offer ursodeoxycholic acid and oral vitamin K
    D Offer ursodeoxycholic acid and discuss elective induction after 37 weeks
    E Offer ursodeoxycholic acid alone

15. A 24-year-old woman presents to the A&E with a 10-hour history of right iliac fossa pain and vaginal bleeding. A urine pregnancy test is positive, and a transvaginal ultrasound reveals a 23 mm adnexal mass with no visible foetal heart beat within the right fallopian tube. Her serum β-hCG is 5200 IU/L. She has no significant past medical history and is keen to avoid surgery if possible. What is the most appropriate treatment option?

    A Expectant management for 24 hours
    B Intravaginal misoprostol
    C Oral mifepristone followed by intravaginal misoprostol
    D Intramuscular methotrexate
    E Salpingectomy

16. A 22-year-old woman, who gave birth 2 weeks ago, presents to her GP complaining of ongoing vaginal bleeding. At first it was heavy and bright red but has recently become brown. She adds that the bleeding appears to worsen when she breastfeeds, and she experiences some mild abdominal pain. Abdominal examination is normal and vaginal examination reveals dark brown blood without clots. What is the most likely diagnosis?

    A Retained products of conception
    B Lochia
    C Endometritis
    D Return of menstruation
    E Placental accreta

17. An 82-year-old woman has returned to the urogynaecology clinic with ongoing complaints of urinary incontinence. She first presented with urinary frequency and urgency, resulting in a few 'accidents'. She has completed 6 weeks of bladder retraining and has seen no improvement in her symptoms. She has a past medical history of type 2 diabetes mellitus and suffered a fractured neck of femur after a fall 6 months ago. What is the most appropriate next step in her management?

    A Tolterodine
    B Oxybutynin
    C Pelvic floor muscle training
    D Mirabegron
    E Percutaneous tibial nerve stimulation

18. A 39-year-old woman, who is 40 weeks' pregnant, is in the active second stage of labour and has become exhausted after 1 hour of pushing. On examination, the cervix is 10 cm dilated and the foetus is in an OP position. The membranes have ruptured, and the head is at the level of the ischial spines. An epidural catheter is *in situ* and the CTG is normal. She has two other children, who were both born by uncomplicated vaginal delivery. How should this patient be managed?

    A Neville Barnes forceps
    B Ventouse delivery
    C Category 1 caesarean section
    D Category 2 caesarean section
    E Category 3 caesarean section

19. A 25-year-old woman presents to her GP complaining of vaginal itching and white curd-like discharge. On speculum examination, a thick white discharge is observed but her vulva appears normal. She has not been sexually active in 6 months and has otherwise been feeling well. After providing advice on lifestyle modification and trigger avoidance, what is the next most appropriate management of this patient?

    A Clotrimazole cream
    B Oral fluconazole
    C Oral fluconazole followed by 6 months of clotrimazole cream
    D Podophyllotoxin cream
    E Oral metronidazole

20. A 28-year-old woman, who is 12 weeks' pregnant, has presented to discuss the results of the blood test performed at her booking visit. She has no past medical history and has not had any problems during the current pregnancy aside from some morning sickness. She is taking folic acid and vitamin D supplements. The blood test results are shown in the following:

Hb: 101 g/L (115–160)
MCV: 106 fL (82–100)
Platelets: 36×10^9/L (150–400)
WBC: 11.6×10^9/L (4–11)
Neutrophils: 7.8×10^9/L (2–7)
Lymphocytes: 2.4×10^9/L (1–3)

What is the most likely diagnosis?

    A Iron deficiency anaemia
    B Microangiopathic haemolytic anaemia
    C HELLP syndrome
    D Idiopathic thrombocytopaenic purpura
    E Gestational thrombocytopaenia

21. A 23-year-old woman presents to A&E with light vaginal bleeding. Her last menstrual period was 8 weeks ago, and a pregnancy test produces a positive result. No intrauterine or extrauterine pregnancy is seen on transvaginal ultrasound scan. Her serum β-hCG is 746 IU/L. She returns two days later and the serum β-hCG is 1540 IU/L. What is the most likely diagnosis?

    A Intrauterine pregnancy
    B Ectopic pregnancy
    C Threatened miscarriage
    D Incomplete miscarriage
    E Molar pregnancy

22. A 29-year-old woman who is 8 weeks' pregnant attends her booking visit. A midstream urine sample is taken which demonstrates the presence of *Escherichia coli*. She denies experiencing any urinary symptoms. What is the most appropriate management option?

    A Nitrofurantoin
    B Trimethoprim
    C Doxycycline
    D Repeat MSU at 36 weeks
    E No treatment necessary

23. A 52-year-old female has had a large loop excision of the transformation zone after cervical intraepithelial neoplasia type ll was identified after colposcopy and biopsy. Which of the following best describes how this patient should be followed up?

    A Repeat smear in 3 years
    B Repeat smear in 5 years
    C Repeat smear in 6 months
    D Repeat colposcopy in 6 months
    E Repeat colposcopy in 1 year

24. A 24-year-old primiparous woman is feeling anxious about the pain that she will experience during childbirth. She has opted to have an induced vaginal delivery with epidural anaesthesia and would like to know more about potential complications. Which of the following is a complication of epidural anaesthesia?

    A Urinary retention
    B Hydrocephalus
    C Hypertension
    D Neonatal tachypnoea
    E Limb spasticity

25. A 51-year-old woman has been suffering from night sweats and hot flushes for the last 6 months. She has found these symptoms deeply embarrassing and it has had a detrimental effect on her mood. She would like to see an improvement in her symptoms, however, she is reluctant to receive hormonal treatment. What is the most appropriate treatment option?

    A Mirabegron
    B Terbutaline
    C Alendronate
    D Fluoxetine
    E Clomiphene

26. A 24-year-old woman, who is 8 weeks' pregnant with her first baby, attends her booking visit. She is found to have a BMI of 36 kg/m². After providing dietary and exercise advice, how else should this patient be managed?

    A Aim to lose weight and achieve a healthy BMI
    B Take 150 mg aspirin daily from 12 weeks' gestation
    C Take 400 *µ*g folate daily from now
    D Recommend orlistat
    E Ensure that she is assessed by an obstetric anaesthetist

27. A 16-year-old girl from Somalia is being investigated for recurrent urinary tract infections. On examination, the doctor notices that her clitoris and labia minora have been surgically removed. The introitus is intact. When questioned, she refuses to answer and attempts to leave clinic. How should this patient be managed?

    A Arrange de-infibulation
    B Arrange clitoral reconstruction
    C Arrange female genital cosmetic surgery
    D Report to the police and child safeguarding team
    E Report to the child safeguarding team only

28. A 41-year-old woman, who is 9 weeks' pregnant, attends her dating scan. A monochorionic diamniotic pregnancy is identified. How should this patient be followed up?

    A Foetal ultrasound assessment every 2 weeks from 20+0 weeks until delivery
    B Foetal ultrasound assessment every 4 weeks from 20+0 weeks until delivery
    C Foetal ultrasound assessment every 2 weeks from 16+0 weeks until delivery
    D Foetal ultrasound assessment every 2 weeks from 16+0 weeks until 26+0 weeks
    E Foetal ultrasound assessment every 4 weeks from 16+0 weeks until 26+0 weeks

29. A 44-year-old woman presents to her GP complaining that, since her caesarean section 6 weeks ago, urine has been continuously leaking out of her vagina and she is having to wear incontinence pads. She denies any dysuria or urgency, but the leakage worsens if she sneezes or coughs. What is the most likely diagnosis?

    A Stress incontinence
    B Urge incontinence
    C Overflow incontinence
    D Cystourethrocele
    E Vesicovaginal fistula

30. A 38-year-old woman is currently in the second stage of labour at 39 weeks' gestation. On vaginal examination, a diamond-shaped depression is palpated anteriorly, and a Y-shaped depression is palpated posteriorly to the right of the pubic symphysis. What is the most likely foetal position?

    A Occipito-anterior
    B Left occipito-posterior
    C Right occipito-posterior
    D Left occipito-transverse
    E Right occipito-transverse

Answers

1. E

Miscarriage is the most common complication of early pregnancy with 1 in 5 pregnancies ending in miscarriage. The cause of miscarriage is usually undetermined but when a cause is found, it is most commonly due to a chromosomal abnormality within the genetic make-up of the conceptus. Recurrent miscarriage is defined as the loss of 3 or more consecutive pregnancies before 24 weeks' gestation. As this patient has only had two previous miscarriages, she would not need further investigation at this stage. The main causes of recurrent miscarriage include antiphospholipid syndrome, balanced translocations within the genomes of the expecting parents, uterine anomalies, and thrombophilia. Based on the likely causes, the following investigations are often used when investigating recurrent miscarriage: transvaginal ultrasound scan (uterine anomalies), coagulation screen (thrombophilia), lupus anticoagulant and anti-cardiolipin antibodies (anti-phospholipid syndrome), and cytogenetic analysis of the patient and partner (balanced translocations). It is worth noting that, often, a cause of recurrent miscarriage will not be identified.

2. C

At the booking visit, all pregnant women should be offered screening for hepatitis B, HIV, and syphilis. With hepatitis B and HIV, treatments can be initiated to reduce the risk of transmission to the neonate. Syphilis, although relatively rare in the UK, is screened as it is associated with miscarriage, stillbirth, and congenital syphilis (characterised by skeletal abnormalities, hepatosplenomegaly, and rhinitis). It can be easily treated by administering IM benzathine penicillin. Rubella infection during the first 20 weeks of pregnancy can cause congenital rubella syndrome, which is characterised by a triad of cataracts, cardiac abnormalities, and sensorineural deafness. Rubella screening has been discontinued since 2016 due to its very low prevalence resulting from the introduction of the MMR vaccine. Women who are not protected against rubella during pregnancy should be offered the MMR vaccine after pregnancy.

3. A

Premenstrual syndrome (PMS) is a term used to describe the symptoms that women can experience in the weeks leading up to their period. The most common symptoms of PMS include mood swings, difficulty sleeping, abdominal pain, breast tenderness, and headaches. PMS is mainly a clinical diagnosis, however, a symptom diary for two cycles may be recommended before commencing treatment to better characterise its severity.

If PMS is mild and has no impact on personal, social or professional life, lifestyle advice alone (regarding diet, exercise, sleep, smoking, and alcohol) is sufficient to improve the symptoms. The patient in this SBA has described some impact of the symptoms on her performance at school and, therefore, this should be considered as moderate PMS. The 1st line treatment option for moderate PMS is the combined oral contraceptive pill (COCP). Alternatives, especially if pain is the predominant symptom, include paracetamol and NSAIDs. If the patient describes significant issues with her mood, cognitive behavioural therapy (CBT) can be considered. Severe PMS, characterised by withdrawal from social and professional activities which prevents normal functioning, can also be treated using the COCP, simple analgesia, and CBT, however, selective serotonin reuptake inhibitors (SSRI) such as fluoxetine may also be considered. SSRIs in this circumstance, may be used continuously or only during the luteal phase of the menstrual cycle.

4. C

Lactational mastitis is a common postpartum condition in which the breast tissue becomes inflamed and painful as a result of an infection. The most common causative organisms are *Staphylococcus* and *Streptococcus*. Patients typically present with breast tenderness and pain. The patient may also develop systemic features of infection such as a fever and malaise. The infection usually becomes established due to stasis of milk resulting from inadequate removal. Therefore, the first step is to recommend continuation of breastfeeding to adequately drain the breast. It will not cause any harm to the baby. If the symptoms do not improve after 12–24 hours of effective milk removal, nipple fissures are present, or the patient is systemically unwell, a 10–14 day course of flucloxacillin should be started.

If a tender mass is palpable and the patient is suffering from swinging fevers, a breast abscess may have developed, which would require incision and drainage. Nipple thrush is another common condition caused by *Candida* infection of the nipples. It presents with pain in the nipples after feeds and creamy white spots may be seen on the palate of the baby. The mother should be treated with topical miconazole and the baby should receive oral nystatin.

5. A

Call–Exner bodies are eosinophilic fluid-filled spaces that are found between granulosa cells and they are pathognomonic of granulosa cell tumours. This is a rare type of ovarian cancer that has a peak incidence in pre-pubertal girls and post-menopausal women. Granulosa cell tumours are one of the five types of sex cord stromal tumours and they secrete oestrogen. This results in symptoms such as post-menopausal bleeding, precocious puberty in young girls, and an increased risk of endometrial cancer. They are treated with conservative surgery but have a high rate of recurrence.

Sertoli–Leydig cell tumours are a rarer subtype of sex cord stromal tumours which mostly affect young women. They produce androgens, resulting in hirsutism, amenorrhoea, and virilisation. Fibromas also belong to the class of sex cord stromal tumours but are benign and tend to affect middle-aged women. They are generally asymptomatic, but a small proportion of cases present with Meigs syndrome (associated with ascites and pleural effusion). A Krukenberg tumour is a metastatic ovarian tumour, most commonly from a primary cancer in the colon or stomach. Dysgerminomas are the most common subtype of malignant germ cell tumour. They tend to affect young girls, are mostly asymptomatic, and are associated with hypercalcaemia and excess β-hCG production.

6. C

Gestational diabetes is the development of diabetes during pregnancy. It is an important antenatal complication that should be promptly diagnosed and managed as it is associated with maternal complications (hypertensive disease in pregnancy, traumatic delivery, and stillbirth) and foetal complications (macrosomia, neonatal hypoglycaemia, and congenital anomalies). Patients are usually diagnosed after having a fasting blood glucose test or OGTT following the detection of glycosuria on a urine dipstick. In patients with a history of previous gestational diabetes, an OGTT should be conducted as soon as possible after the booking visit. Similarly, in patients with risk factors for gestational diabetes, an OGTT should be offered at 24–28 weeks.

A 2-hour OGTT greater than 7.8 mmol/L or a fasting blood glucose level greater than 5.6 mmol/L is diagnostic of gestational diabetes. Once diagnosed, the 1st line management option is dietary modification and exercise. If this fails to achieve target blood glucose levels after 1–2 weeks, metformin should be added. If this also fails to achieve satisfactory blood glucose levels, insulin should be added. Patients with a fasting blood glucose level greater than 7 mmol/L at diagnosis should begin treatment immediately with insulin. Patients with a fasting blood glucose of 6–6.9 mmol/L with evidence of complications should also be treated with insulin. Glibenclamide is a sulphonylurea that can be used as an alternative if metformin is not tolerated. Patients should be seen regularly at an antenatal diabetes clinic.

Patients should be taught how to monitor their capillary glucose levels and they should aim for the following blood glucose targets:

- Fasting <5.3 mmol/L
- 1 hour post-meal <7.8 mmol/L
- 2 hours post-meal <6.4 mmol/L

The management of gestational diabetes is summarised in the following RevChart.

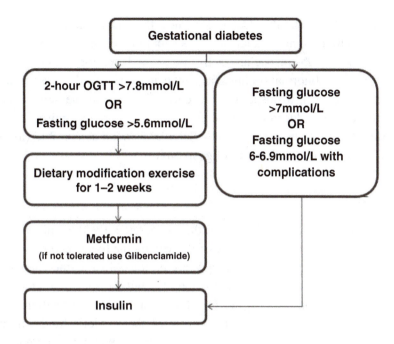

7. B

Failing to conceive after 1 year of regular unprotected sexual intercourse warrants further investigation. All women should have a mid-luteal progesterone measurement (taken 7 days before the first day of a period) to confirm that she is ovulating. A chlamydia screen should also be requested as it can cause subfertility. Other tests may be requested if clinically indicated (summarised as follows).

Test	Indication
Serum progesterone	Prolonged irregular periods (confirm ovulation)
Serum gonadotrophins (FSH and LH)	Irregular cycles (if hypogonadotrophic hypogonadism or polycystic ovarian syndrome is suspected)
Thyroid function tests	Suspected thyroid disease
Serum prolactin	Galactorrhoea or suspected pituitary tumour
Basal body temperature	Does not reliably predict ovulation so is not recommended

The male partner should also be screened for chlamydia and a semen sample should be sent for analysis. This should be collected after at least 2 days of sexual abstinence and delivered to the laboratory within 1 hour of production. Abnormal findings on semen analysis include oligospermia (low sperm count), azoospermia (absence of sperm in the semen) and asthenospermia (reduced motility). If abnormalities are recognised, a second sample should be sent 3 months later or as soon as possible (in the case of azoospermia and severe oligospermia).

8. A

Amniotic fluid is a protective liquid that is secreted into the amniotic sac by the amnion and the foetus. It is swallowed by the foetus and most of it will be absorbed, entering the foetal circulation. Most of the fluid will then pass through the placenta but some of it will return to the amniotic sac by transudation through the foetal skin or by foetal urination. The amniotic fluid index (AFI) is an estimate of the amniotic fluid volume measured from the deepest pocket of four uterine quadrants. The normal range for AFI varies with gestational age, but an AFI between 5 and 25 cm is considered normal between 20 and 35 weeks (after which the amniotic fluid volume decreases).

Polyhydramnios describes excess accumulation of amniotic fluid and is defined by an AFI greater than 25 cm. Risks of polyhydramnios include preterm delivery, cord prolapse, placental abruption, and malpresentation. Mechanisms and causes of polyhydramnios are listed in the following table.

Mechanism	Cause
Increased foetal urine production	Maternal cardiac or renal disease Maternal diabetes mellitus Multiple pregnancy Hydrops fetalis
Inability of the foetus to swallow or absorb amniotic fluid	Neurological or muscular abnormality (e.g. myotonic dystrophy, anencephaly) Foetal gastrointestinal obstruction (e.g. duodenal atresia) Chromosomal abnormalities (e.g. Down syndrome)
Idiopathic	30–50% of cases

Oligohydramnios is a deficiency of amniotic fluid and is defined as an AFI less than 5 cm. Risks include stillbirth, limb contractures, and incomplete lung maturation. Mechanisms and causes are listed in the following table.

Mechanism	Cause
Leakage of amniotic fluid	Rupture of membranes
Reduced foetal urine production	Post-dates pregnancy
	Renal tract malformations or renal failure
	Foetal urinary obstruction (e.g. posterior urethral valve)
	Intrauterine growth restriction
Other	Pre-eclampsia

9. D

The progesterone-only pill is a useful option for patients in whom oestrogen-based contraceptives are contraindicated. The progesterone-only pill works by thickening cervical mucus, thereby preventing the entry of sperm into the uterus. All progesterone-based contraceptives will cause some degree of thickening of the cervical mucus, however, the primary mechanism of action of the progesterone implant and injection is inhibition of ovulation. As the progesterone-only pill takes 2 days to sufficiently thicken cervical mucus to prevent the passage of sperm, additional contraceptive measures should be taken for the first 2 days after starting the pill.

The copper IUD and levonorgestrel IUS works by thinning the endometrium and preventing implantation. The copper IUD also has a spermicidal effect. Combined hormonal methods (e.g. pill, patch, and ring) and emergency contraception works by preventing ovulation.

10. B

Umbilical cord prolapse is usually diagnosed when the umbilical cord is palpated below the presenting part of the foetal head after rupture of membranes. It causes acute compromise of the foetal circulation resulting from vasospasm of the umbilical vessels. This can cause foetal hypoxia and produce pathological features on a CTG (e.g. foetal bradycardia). Risk factors of cord prolapse include preterm labour, foetal malpresentation, polyhydramnios, low birth weight, and artificial rupture of membranes.

Caesarean section is the recommended mode of delivery in most cases of cord prolapse when vaginal birth is not imminent. A category 1 caesarean section (within 30 minutes) is required if there is a suspicious or pathological CTG. A category 2 caesarean section (within 60–75 minutes) may be considered if the foetal heart pattern is normal, but continuous CTG monitoring is essential and if the CTG becomes abnormal, category 1 caesarean section should be considered. Whilst awaiting an emergency caesarean section, the presenting part should be elevated either manually or by filling the bladder to elevate the cord and reduce cord compression. There should be minimal handling of the cord to prevent vasospasm. Cord compression can be further reduced by the mother adopting the knee-to-chest or left lateral position. If the patient is fully dilated, instrumental delivery may be considered if it can be done safely and quickly. McRoberts manoeuvre with suprapubic pressure is a crucial step in the management of shoulder dystocia.

11. B

Polycystic ovarian syndrome (PCOS) is a complex but common condition characterised by oligoovulation/anovulation, clinical or biochemical features of hyperandrogenism and polycystic ovaries on ultrasound ($\geq$20 in one or both ovaries measuring 2–9 mm in diameter). The Rotterdam criteria states that two of the three aforementioned features are necessary to diagnose PCOS. Other typical features of PCOS include insulin resistance, subfertility, and weight gain. It is estimated that around 10% of females of reproductive age have PCOS, although many will be unaware of the condition. A transvaginal ultrasound scan to demonstrate the presence of multiple cysts on the ovaries will help confirm the diagnosis of PCOS. Mid-luteal progesterone is also useful to demonstrate anovulation, however, this is not specific to PCOS. An elevated LH:FSH ratio (more than 1:1) may also be seen in PCOS.

There is no cure for PCOS, although symptoms tend to improve considerably after the menopause. Management of PCOS depends on which aspect of the condition is most troublesome to the patient. For example, patients who present complaining of irregular bleeding can be managed by using the combined oral contraceptive pill to control the bleeding. On the other hand, a patient, like the one in this SBA, who is hoping to get pregnant should be managed by recommending weight loss and clomiphene citrate (selective oestrogen receptor modulator that stimulates ovulation).

12. C

According to NICE, the indications for a planned caesarean section are:

- Pregnant women with a singleton breech presentation at term, for whom external cephalic version is contraindicated or has been unsuccessful.
- Multiple pregnancy, if the first twin is not cephalic at the time of planned birth.
- Women with placenta praevia in which the placenta partly or completely covers the internal cervical os.
- Women with a suspected morbidly adherent placenta.
- Women with HIV who are not receiving anti-retroviral therapy or are receiving anti-retroviral therapy and have a viral load of 400 copies/mL or more.
- Women who are co-infected with hepatitis C and HIV.
- Women with primary genital herpes simplex infection occurring in the third trimester of pregnancy.

There are two types of surgical technique used for caesarean section: the classical section (involving a longitudinal midline incision) and the lower uterine segment section (involving a transverse incision superior to the edge of the bladder). Classical caesarean sections are now rarely performed due to the risk of haemorrhage and uterine rupture. As a result, the Royal College of Obstetricians and Gynaecologists recommends planned caesarean section in women with previous uterine rupture or a classical caesarean scar.

13. C

Endometrial hyperplasia develops under the influence of oestrogenic stimulation. Excess oestrogen exposure can come from an endogenous source, such as oestrogen-producing tumours and anovulatory cycles (e.g. polycystic ovarian syndrome), or an exogenous source, such as oestrogen-only hormone replacement therapy, tamoxifen, and early menarche/late menopause. Reduced endogenous progesterone production also increases the risk of endometrial hyperplasia and progesterone is high during pregnancy so nulliparous women are at increased risk of endometrial hyperplasia. Other risk factors include age, obesity, type 2 diabetes mellitus, and genetic conditions (e.g. hereditary non-polyposis colorectal cancer).

Interestingly, smoking is a protective factor for endometrial cancer as are parity and the combined oral contraceptive (due to the effect of progesterone). The combined oral contraceptive pill also has a protective effect against ovarian cancer but is associated with an increased risk of breast and cervical cancer.

14. D

Obstetric cholestasis is a condition that typically occurs in the 3rd trimester of pregnancy and is characterised by an interruption in the flow of bile that resolves after delivery. It is associated with an increased risk of stillbirth, preterm delivery, and meconium passage. Patients with obstetric cholestasis may be offered ursodeoxycholic acid (UDCA) as it was thought to reduce itching and improve liver function, however, the latest evidence suggests that UDCA does not cause a significant improvement in symptoms or outcomes. Given the risks, a discussion should take place with the mother regarding induction of labour after 37 weeks' gestation. As stillbirth associated with obstetric cholestasis cannot be reliably predicted or prevented by monitoring, the benefits of delivery at 37 weeks' gestation outweighs the risks. Patients with severe obstetric cholestasis (bile acids greater than 40 μmol/L) should be offered elective delivery at 36 weeks.

Topical emollients (e.g. calamine lotion) are safe to use and may provide temporary relief of symptoms. Cholestyramine is a bile acid chelating agent which improves pruritus but is generally not recommended as it is usually poorly tolerated with little data to support its use. Antihistamines (e.g. chlorphenamine) can be helpful if the itching is disturbing sleep as it has a mild sedating effect. Obstetric cholestasis can reduce the absorption of dietary fats due to failure of excretion of bile into the gastrointestinal tract. Vitamin K is a fat-soluble vitamin that is required for the production of coagulation factors II, VII, IX, and X. Therefore, daily vitamin K is recommended in women with obstetric cholestasis who have a prolonged clotting time.

15. E

An ectopic pregnancy is defined as the implantation of a pregnancy outside the uterine cavity. They are most commonly found within the ampulla of the fallopian tube. Ectopic pregnancies must be managed promptly as they could otherwise cause considerable damage to surrounding structures or they could rupture resulting in peritonism. Ectopic pregnancies can be treated expectantly, medically, or surgically depending on the presence of symptoms, serum β-hCG, size of the adnexal mass, and past medical history.

Expectant management relies on the premise that a significant proportion of ectopic pregnancies will resolve without treatment. It is only considered if serum β-hCG is less than 1000 IU/L, the patient is stable and asymptomatic, and no foetal heartbeat is detected. This involves taking serial β-hCG measurements until levels become undetectable.

Medical management with intramuscular methotrexate is considered if all of the following criteria are fulfilled:

- Serum β-hCG <1500 IU/L
- No significant pain
- Unruptured ectopic pregnancy with adnexal mass <35 mm with no visible heartbeat

A surgical approach is preferred if any of the following criteria are fulfilled:

- Serum β-hCG >5000 IU/L
- Significant pain
- Adnexal mass >35 mm
- Visible foetal heartbeat

A choice of medical or surgical management can be offered if β-hCG is 1500–5000 IU/L. A laparoscopic salpingectomy (removal of the affected fallopian tube) is the preferred option in most cases, however, salpingotomy (removal of the affected portion of the fallopian tube with anastomosis of the loose ends) may be considered in patients with risk factors for subfertility (e.g. previous pelvic inflammatory disease or tubal damage). Salpingotomy is a less definitive treatment option and 1 in 5 patients will require further treatment.

Intravaginal misoprostol is used in the medical management of miscarriage. Oral mifepristone and intravaginal misoprostol are used together in the medical termination of pregnancy.

The management of ectopic pregnancy is summarised in the following RevChart.

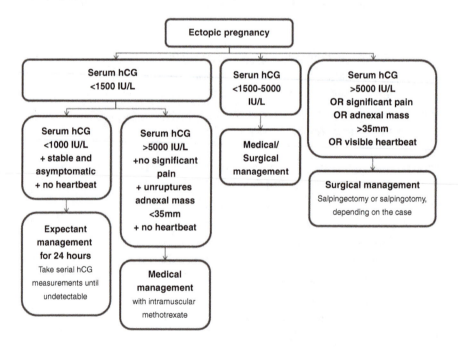

16. B

Lochia is vaginal discharge consisting of blood, mucus, and uterine tissue that occurs for up to 4–6 weeks following delivery. The bleeding is initially heavy, bright red, and may contact clots. Over a matter of weeks, it gradually becomes dark brown and lighter. The bleeding may become heavier when breastfeeding, as a neuroendocrine reflex arc stimulates the uterus to contract. This may be accompanied by crampy period-like pain. The patient should be reassured that this is a normal process, however, they should be discouraged from using tampons as this increases the risk of infection.

Endometritis is inflammation of the endometrium which occurs when an infection ascends through the cervix during or after childbirth. Factors that increase the risk of endometritis include prolonged rupture of membranes, prolonged labour, caesarean delivery, and postpartum haemorrhage. Infection tends to be polymicrobial (predominantly group B streptococci and gram-negative anaerobes). Endometritis is the most common cause of secondary postpartum haemorrhage and typically presents within the first 2–3 days with malodourous blood discharge, lower abdominal pain, uterine tenderness, and fever. It is treated using IV broad-spectrum antibiotics (e.g. co-amoxiclav). Endometritis may be caused by retained products of conception, which refers to the persistence of placental or foetal tissue in the uterus following delivery. Retained products may present with features of endometritis and a poorly contracted, boggy uterus. Placenta accreta is a condition in which the placenta attaches abnormally to the wall of the uterus. It carries a high risk of retained products of conception, as the placenta often fails to detach fully from the uterus.

17. D

This patient has presented with features suggestive of urge incontinence and has completed the 1st line management (6 weeks of bladder retraining) with no improvement in her symptoms. The next step in managing urge incontinence involves offering a bladder stabilising drug — usually an antimuscarinic such as tolterodine, darifenacin, or oxybutynin.

However, antimuscarinics should be avoided in frail, elderly women as it increases their risk of falls. As this woman has already suffered a fractured neck of femur as a result of a fall, an alternative medication should be sought. In this case, mirabegron, a β_3-agonist, would be a useful option. If mirabegron also fails to resolve the symptoms, surgical procedures such as botox injections, percutaneous tibial nerve stimulation, and sacral nerve stimulation may be considered. Pelvic floor muscular training is the 1st line treatment option for stress incontinence. It aims to reduce the symptoms by strengthening the pelvic floor muscles, which are responsible for maintaining the integrity of the bladder outlet.

The management of urge incontinence is summarised in the following RevChart.

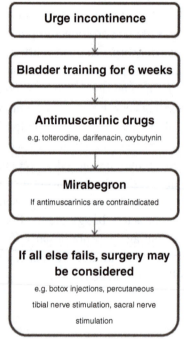

18. B

This patient is experiencing a prolonged second stage of labour defined as an active second stage lasting more than 1 hour in multiparous woman and more than 2 hours in nulliparous women. The delay in this case may be because of the occipito-posterior position of the foetus. Delayed second stage is an indication for instrumental delivery with either forceps or ventouse. The choice of instrument depends on the clinical circumstances and operator experience. However, since rotation of the foetus is required, ventouse delivery is appropriate in this case. This involves attaching a suction cup to the head and applying traction to rotate the foetus. Neville Barnes forceps do not allow rotation and can only be used for occipito-anterior positions. The requirements for delivery with Neville Barnes forceps can be remembered with the mnemonic **FORCEPS**: **F**ully dilated, **O**ccipito-anterior position, **R**uptured membranes, **C**ephalic presentation, **E**ngaged presenting part, adequate **P**ain relief, and **S**phincter (empty bladder). Kielland forceps are rotational forceps that can turn the baby to an occipito-anterior position but are rarely used due to the risk of perineal tears and need for episiotomy.

A caesarean section may be necessary if instrumental delivery is unsuccessful after three attempts or if the CTG reveals signs of foetal distress. There are four categories of caesarean section: category 1 (immediate threat to life of women or foetus), category 2 (no immediate threat to life), category 3 (requires early delivery), and category 4 (at a time that suits the woman and maternity service). Category 1 should ideally be performed within 30 minutes and category 2 within 60–75 minutes.

19. A

Vulvovaginal candidiasis can be classified as uncomplicated or complicated. An uncomplicated infection is sporadic or infrequent, mild-moderate, caused by *Candida albicans* or not associated with risk factors (e.g. pregnancy, diabetes, steroid treatment). A complicated infection may be recurrent (four or more episodes in one year), severe, caused by yeasts other than *Candida albicans* or associated with risk factors. This classification determines the type of treatment that is necessary. For uncomplicated infections, women are prescribed an intravaginal antifungal cream or pessary (such as clotrimazole). If there are vulval symptoms, a topical imidazole (clotrimazole or ketoconazole) is prescribed in addition to an oral or intravaginal antifungal. This patient has an uncomplicated infection without vulval involvement, so clotrimazole cream is the most appropriate treatment. Patients with candidiasis should also be advised to avoid predisposing factors (e.g. washing the vulva excessively with soap). Patients should instead use a soap substitute (e.g. emollient) and consider using probiotics.

Oral fluconazole is used for severe *Candida* infections and uncomplicated infections in women aged over 60 years, as patients in this age group tend to prefer an oral route of administration. Recurrent infections are treated with an induction course of oral fluconazole or an intravaginal antifungal followed by a maintenance regimen of 6 months' treatment with an oral or intravaginal antifungal. Oral antifungals should be avoided in pregnancy. Metronidazole is an antibiotic used to treat trichomoniasis and bacterial vaginosis, and podophyllotoxin is used to treat anogenital warts.

20. D

Idiopathic thrombocytopaenic purpura (ITP) is a condition in which platelets are destroyed by autoantibodies directed against platelet antigens. Platelet count does tend to drop by around 10% in most pregnancies (known as gestational thrombocytopaenia) although the mechanism is poorly understood. Gestational thrombocytopaenia tends to be asymptomatic and the platelet count will rarely drop below 70×10^9/L. Although it can be difficult to distinguish between gestational thrombocytopaenia and ITP, a platelet count as low as 36×10^9/L is much more likely to be ITP. Furthermore, ITP tends to occur in the first trimester whereas gestational thrombocytopaenia tends to occur in the third trimester. ITP should be identified and treated promptly using steroids as the autoantibodies can cross the placenta causing neonatal thrombocytopaenia, which can increase the risk of intracranial haemorrhage. If there is no response to steroids or the platelet count is very low, IVIG may be used. It is important to be aware of the platelet count at term as it can have implications on the delivery. A platelet count of more than 70×10^9/L is necessary for an epidural and more than 50×10^9/L is necessary for a safe delivery.

Iron deficiency anaemia would cause a microcytic anaemia. Furthermore, a decrease in haemoglobin and a rise in MCV is expected in pregnancy. Microangiopathic haemolytic anaemia is likely to cause a more profound anaemia and would not have such a major impact on platelet count. She is only at 12 weeks' gestation and there is no evidence of elevated liver enzymes or haemolysis so HELLP syndrome is unlikely.

21. A

This patient has a pregnancy of unknown location (PUL), which is defined as a positive pregnancy test with no intrauterine or extrauterine pregnancy visible on transvaginal ultrasound scan. In PUL, two serum β-hCG measurements should be taken 48 hours apart to determine the subsequent management. A very low initial reading may indicate miscarriage. If β-hCG increases by more than 63% after 48 hours, the patient is likely to have a developing intrauterine pregnancy and a transvaginal ultrasound should be offered 7–14 days later to determine the location of the pregnancy. Intrauterine pregnancies are not usually visible on transvaginal ultrasound until the serum β-hCG exceeds 1000 IU/L.

An earlier scan can be considered if the serum β-hCG level is equal to or greater than 1500 IU/L because, at this level, a pregnancy should be visible on ultrasound so a scan is needed as an ectopic pregnancy cannot be ruled out. If the β-hCG decreases by more than 50% after 48 hours, the patient has most likely had a miscarriage. She should be advised to take a urine pregnancy test 14 days later and, if the test is positive, she should return to the early pregnancy assessment service for further investigation. If the pregnancy test is negative, no further action is required. If the serum β-hCG decreases by less than 50% or increases by less than 63%, the patient may have an ectopic pregnancy and needs to be seen in the early pregnancy assessment service within 24 hours. The early pregnancy assessment service provides transvaginal ultrasound scans to locate the pregnancy and determine whether there is a foetal pole and heartbeat.

22. A

The midstream urine (MSU) sample taken at the booking visit aims to detect asymptomatic bacteriuria. This is a condition characterised by the presence of clinically significant amounts of bacteria in the urine in the absence of symptoms. Asymptomatic bacteriuria is associated with an increased risk of preterm delivery and pyelonephritis during pregnancy, so treatment is recommended. It is usually treated with a 7-day course of nitrofurantoin. Alternative options include amoxicillin and cephalexin. Trimethoprim is contraindicated in the first 12 weeks of pregnancy as it is a folate antagonist and can increase the risk of neural tube defects. Doxycycline belongs to the tetracycline class of antibiotics. Tetracyclines are contraindicated in pregnancy and in young children as it has some teratogenic effects, including issues with the formation of bones and teeth.

23. C

During colposcopy, a speculum is inserted into the vagina and a colposcope (specialised microscope) which allows direct visualisation of the cervix. 5% acetic acid (which turns dysplastic areas white) and Lugol's iodine (which turns normal cervical epithelium brown) are applied. If there are obvious abnormal cells in the cervix, they can be removed at the point-of-care via large loop excision of the transformation zone (LLETZ). This involves excising the abnormal cells using a heated wire under local anaesthetic. The tissue removed is sent for histological analysis and confirmation of a clear excision margin. Patients undergoing a LLETZ should be reassured that it does not affect fertility. If abnormal cells are not obvious during colposcopy, a directed punch biopsy is taken and sent for histological analysis. If CIN 1 is found on biopsy, the patient should be offered a repeat smear in 12 months to check for resolution. If CIN ll or CIN lll is found, the patient will be referred for colposcopy and the abnormal tissue will be removed by LLETZ or cone biopsy.

After receiving treatment for CIN via LLETZ or cone biopsy, the patient should be followed up with a repeat smear 6 months later, including human papilloma virus (HPV) testing. If HPV is negative, the patient can return to routine cervical screening. If HPV is positive or moderate or severe dyskaryosis is found, they should be referred for colposcopy.

24. A

Epidural anaesthesia is regularly used on the labour ward and is an effective form of pain relief. It involves inserting a catheter through the gap between two lumbar vertebrae and into the epidural space. A solution that usually contains a local anaesthetic (e.g. bupivacaine) and an opioid (e.g. fentanyl) can be instilled via the catheter. Although epidural anaesthesia is often effective at controlling pain, it can have several adverse effects which require close monitoring. Blockage of the output to the bladder from the spinal cord can lead to patients losing the sensation of needing to urinate, which can result in urinary retention. If patients fail to produce an adequate volume of urine, a urinary catheter may be inserted.

Hypotension is a common complication as the anaesthetic can block the sympathetic output to peripheral blood vessels leading to widespread vasodilation. Therefore, blood pressure should be monitored whilst a patient is receiving epidural anaesthesia. Accidentally entering the subarachnoid space when performing an epidural may lead to leakage of CSF resulting in a spinal headache. The opioid in the epidural solution could cross into the baby and cause neonatal respiratory depression. Epidural anaesthesia may cause loss of movement and sensation in the legs.

25. D

This patient is predominantly complaining of the vasomotor symptoms of the menopause (hot flushes and night sweats). Although hormone replacement therapy is the preferred treatment option, the patient's reluctance to be treated by hormonal therapy requires exploration of other options. Fluoxetine is a selective serotonin reuptake inhibitor (SSRI) which is commonly used in the treatment of depression. It can also be used to treat the vasomotor symptoms of the menopause. Other non-hormonal treatments that are effective at treating vasomotor symptoms include α-agonists (e.g. clonidine) and β-blockers (e.g. propranolol).

Mirabegron is a β_3 agonist that is used to treat urge incontinence. Terbutaline is a β_2 agonist that is used as a tocolytic in preterm labour. Alendronate is a bisphosphonate that may be used in post-menopausal women to treat or prevent osteoporosis. Clomiphene is a selective oestrogen receptor modulator that is used to stimulate ovulation in women with fertility issues.

26. B

Women with a booking BMI of 30 kg/m^2 or more should be made aware of the risks that obesity poses to themselves and their unborn baby. Obesity in pregnancy is associated with an increased risk of miscarriage, gestational diabetes, pre-eclampsia, venous thromboembolism, macrosomia, and post-partum haemorrhage. Ideally, women should reach a healthy BMI before conception, to reduce the risk of these complications. Dieting and weight loss drugs (e.g. orlistat) are not recommended during pregnancy as it may cause harm to the unborn baby. Instead, women should be advised to eat a healthy, balanced diet, and undertake at least 30 minutes of moderate intensity exercise daily. Examples of appropriate exercises include swimming, brisk walking, or strength conditioning. Many women may believe that they need to eat more to meet the additional demands of the growing foetus, however, energy requirements do not change in the first 6 months of pregnancy and increase moderately in the third trimester. Women with a BMI greater than 30 kg/m^2 should be offered a referral to a dietician. Women with a BMI greater than 40 kg/m^2 should be referred to an obstetric anaesthetist for assessment. This is because these women are more likely to need an instrumental delivery and it may be more difficult to administer epidural anaesthesia. All women who are intending to conceive should be advised to start taking 400 μg of folic acid daily. This should be continued until 12 weeks' gestation. Women with a BMI greater than 30 kg/m^2 should be advised to take 5 mg folic acid instead. This patient would also benefit from receiving 150 mg aspirin from 12 weeks' gestation until 36 weeks' gestation to prevent pre-eclampsia as she has more than one of the following moderate risk factors:

- First pregnancy
- Age 40 years or older
- Pregnancy interval of more than 10 years
- BMI of 35 kg/m^2 or more at booking visit
- Family history of pre-eclampsia

27. D

This patient has been a victim of female genital mutilation (FGM). This refers to all procedures involving partial or total removal of the external female genitalia for non-medical reasons. According to the World Health Organization, FGM is classified into one of four types:

- **Type 1:** Partial or total removal of the clitoris and/or the prepuce (skin covering the clitoris).
- **Type 2:** Partial or total removal of the clitoris and the labia minora, with or without excision of the labia majora.
- **Type 3:** Narrowing of the vaginal orifice with creation of a covering seal by cutting and appositioning the labia minora and/or labia majora, with or without excision of the clitoris (infibulation).
- **Type 4:** All other harmful procedures to the female genitalia for non-medical purposes, including pricking, piercing, incising and cauterisation.

According to the Female Genital Mutilation Act 2003, FGM is illegal and it is an offence for those with parental responsibility to fail to protect a girl from FGM. If FGM is confirmed in a girl under 18 years of age, it is mandatory to report it to the police within one month of confirmation. All children with confirmed or suspected FGM should also be seen by child safeguarding services. De-infibulation is a surgical procedure that re-opens the introitus in women with type 3 FGM. The patient in this case has type 2 FGM so de-infibulation is not a viable option. Clitoral reconstruction is not performed because of high complication rates.

28. C

Multiple pregnancies are associated with various antenatal, intrapartum, and foetal complications (listed as follows):

- **Antenatal:** Hyperemesis, anaemia, polyhydramnios, gestational diabetes, pre-eclampsia, and antepartum haemorrhage.

- **Intrapartum:** Malpresentation, cord prolapse, foetal distress, and postpartum haemorrhage.
- **Foetal:** Stillbirth, prematurity, intrauterine growth restriction, malformations, twin-to-twin transfusion syndrome (TTTS), and selective growth restriction (sGR).

TTTS and sGR are specific complications that arise in monochorionic twins only (i.e. sharing one placenta). TTTS arises from abnormal vascular communications in the placenta that connect the two foetal circulations resulting in excess blood flow from one twin (donor) to the other (recipient). If the twins are diamniotic (i.e. different amniotic sacs), polyhydramnios in the recipient and oligohydramnios and growth restriction in the donor will be observed. sGR occurs when the placental blood supply between the twins is imbalanced. To monitor for such complications, an uncomplicated monochorionic pregnancy requires ultrasound assessment every 2 weeks from 16 weeks' gestation until delivery. This should involve measuring liquor volume to assess for TTTS and estimated foetal weight to assess for sGR. TTTS presenting before 26 weeks' gestation should be referred to a foetal medicine specialist for treatment with fetoscopic laser ablation of the communicating vessels. Dichorionic pregnancies are considered lower risk than monochorionic pregnancies and so require less intensive monitoring. Ultrasound assessment every four weeks from 20 weeks' gestation until delivery is recommended.

29. E

A vesicovaginal fistula is a subtype of urogenital fistula that extends between the bladder and vault of the vagina and allows continuous involuntary discharge of urine through the vagina. Causes can be divided into acquired or congenital. Acquired causes include obstructed labour, malignancy, gynaecological surgery, radiotherapy, and trauma. Congenital causes are very rare and are often associated with other urogenital malformations. The classic presentation is continuous (day and night) incontinence with a history of obstructed labour or gynaecological surgery. The patient might also complain of a degree of stress incontinence as sneezing or coughing causes an increase in intra-abdominal pressure which pushes more urine through the fistula.

Stress incontinence is the involuntary loss of urine with any action that increases intra-abdominal pressure (e.g. coughing, sneezing, laughing) and does not involve the continuous passage of urine. Urge incontinence is the involuntary leakage of urine that is immediately preceded by a strong desire to pass urine. It is associated with nocturia and increased frequency. Overflow incontinence is the involuntary loss of urine that occurs when there is an obstruction of the bladder outlet (e.g. benign prostatic hyperplasia). The bladder fills and chronic retention causes a loss of the urge to urinate. Overflow incontinence can also result from autonomic neuropathy (e.g. diabetes mellitus) in which there are reduced neural signals from the bladder and a loss of detrusor muscle contraction. It is also associated with several classes of medications including anticholinergic agents and calcium channel blockers. Cystourethrocele is a prolapse of the anterior vaginal wall, involving the bladder and urethra, which presents with stress incontinence, increased urinary frequency, and retention.

30. C

The most anatomically favourable position for the foetal head to pass through the birth canal is occipito-anterior (OA) — facing the mother's back. Occipito-posterior (OP) and occipito-transverse (OT) are types of malposition. Position is assessed on vaginal examination using the anterior fontanelle (diamond-shaped depression) and posterior fontanelle (Y-shaped depression) as landmarks. In the OA position, the anterior fontanelle will be felt posteriorly (relative to the mother) to the posterior fontanelle in a longitudinal plane. The position can be further characterised by describing the relationship of the occiput to the pubic symphysis — either right or left. In this SBA, the anterior fontanelle is felt anteriorly and the posterior fontanelle is felt posteriorly and to the right of the pubic symphysis suggesting that the foetus is in a right occipito-posterior position. Most OP presentations will spontaneously rotate into an OA position as labour progresses, but failure to do so may result in slow progress in the second stage requiring instrumental delivery.

Presentation (not to be confused with *position*) describes the crude foetal body part that enters the maternal pelvis. Cephalic presentation (head down) is the most common and anatomically most favourable. Breech, shoulder, face, and brow are types of malpresentation which can lead to complication in labour.

Obstetrics and Gynaecology: Paper 3

Questions

1. A 36-year-old woman, who is 10 weeks' pregnant, presents to the GUM clinic with green, frothy vaginal discharge. High vaginal swabs identify *Trichomoniasis vaginalis* and Group B *Streptococcus*. A 7-day course of metronidazole is offered. How else should this patient be managed?

   A Treat with antenatal benzylpenicillin only
   B Treat with intrapartum benzylpenicillin only
   C Treat with intrapartum benzylpenicillin and intrapartum vaginal cleansing
   D Treat with antenatal and intrapartum benzylpenicillin
   E No further treatment is necessary

2. A 62-year-old woman returns to the urogynaecology clinic complaining that, despite bladder retaining and a 8-week course of tolterodine, she is still having to use incontinence pads. She is open to discussing invasive procedures and would like to avoid any more medication. Urodynamic studies report detrusor overactivity. What is the next most appropriate step in this patient's management?

    A Urinary diversion
    B Colposuspension
    C Botulinum toxin type A injection
    D Percutaneous sacral nerve stimulation
    E Augmentation cystoplasty

3. Following an uncomplicated caesarean section for multiple pregnancy, a 44-year-old woman suddenly becomes extremely anxious. She is tachypnoeic and tachycardic with a blood pressure of 78/36 mm Hg. Her lips turn blue and her peripheries are cold. She begins to bleed from the caesarean incision site and she goes into cardiac arrest. What is the most likely diagnosis?

    A Eclampsia
    B Uterine inversion
    C Uterine rupture
    D Pulmonary embolism
    E Amniotic fluid embolism

4. A 22-year-old woman presents to the GUM clinic complaining of an itchy and burning vulva. She describes green, frothy discharge, and painful urination. On examination, her vulva and vagina appear inflamed and foul-smelling discharge is observed. A speculum examination reveals punctate haemorrhages on the cervix. What is the most likely diagnosis?

    A Vulvovaginal candidiasis
    B Trichomoniasis
    C Bacterial vaginosis
    D Chlamydia
    E Gonorrhoea

5. A 28-year-old woman, who is 32 weeks' pregnant, presents after experiencing a sudden gush of clear fluid from her vagina. A sterile speculum examination reveals pooling of amniotic fluid and preterm prelabour rupture of membranes is diagnosed. Oral erythromycin is

commenced and a CTG monitor is attached. Antenatal corticosteroids are recommended. Which of the following options is most appropriate?

    A 2 × 24 mg IM betamethasone 12 hours apart
    B 2 × 12 mg IM betamethasone 24 hours apart
    C 2 × 6 mg IM dexamethasone 12 hours apart
    D 2 × 12 mg IM dexamethasone 24 hours apart
    E 2 × 30 mg oral prednisolone 12 hours apart

6. A 30-year-old woman returns to clinic after being diagnosed with endometriosis. She was started on the combined oral contraceptive pill and recommended simple analgesia, but her symptoms have persisted. She does not currently have any plans of getting pregnant, but would like to start a family within the next 5 years. What is the most appropriate management?

    A Laparoscopic hysterectomy
    B Endometrial ablation
    C Laparoscopic excision or ablation plus adhesiolysis
    D Laparoscopic excision followed by hormonal treatment
    E Myomectomy

7. A 32-year-old woman is admitted after experiencing an eclamptic seizure. Her blood pressure is 168/104 mm Hg and IV labetalol is commenced. She is also started on IV magnesium sulphate to prevent further seizures. Which of the following is important to monitor in order to identify magnesium toxicity?

    A Respiratory rate
    B Temperature
    C Blood pressure
    D Cardiotocograph
    E Urine output

8. A 35-year-old woman is being investigated in the fertility clinic. She has had irregular periods for the past 2 years and has been having

regular unprotected sexual intercourse for over 12 months without success. She has two children who were both delivered by caesarean section. She also had a myomectomy for submucosal fibroids 2 years ago. Her blood test results are shown as follows:

FSH: 5 U/L (1.2–9 U/L)
LH: 7 U/L (<14.7 U/L)
TSH: 2.5 mU/L (0–5.7 mU/L)
Prolactin: 150 IU/L (53–360 U/L)
Sex hormone binding globulin: 75 nmol/L (26–110 nmol/L)
Oestradiol: 350 pmol/L (101–905 pmol/L)
Testosterone: 1.8 nmol/L (0.2–2.9 nmol/L)
Midluteal progesterone: 37 nmol/L (>35 nmol/L)
Pregnancy test: Negative

What is the most likely underlying diagnosis?

A Turner syndrome
B Asherman's syndrome
C Kallman syndrome
D Sheehan syndrome
E Polycystic ovarian syndrome

9. During labour, which foetal movement occurs after the foetal head reaches the pelvic floor?

A Internal rotation
B External rotation
C Extension
D Flexion
E Engagement

10. A 67-year-old woman, who was recently diagnosed with endometrial cancer, has had an MRI to stage the cancer. It finds that the cancer has spread to the fallopian tubes, ovaries, uterosacral ligaments, and the parametrium. What FIGO stage is this cancer?

A Stage I
B Stage II
C Stage III
D Stage IV
E Not enough information to determine stage

11. A 27-year-old woman, who is 26 weeks' pregnant, presents to the antenatal clinic after developing several painful sores on her labia. On further questioning, she reveals that she had unprotected sex with a new partner 1 week ago. She has never been pregnant before and would like to have a vaginal delivery. Given the most likely diagnosis, how should her pregnancy be managed hereafter?

A Viral PCR
B Oral aciclovir starting immediately and expectant vaginal delivery
C Oral aciclovir starting at 36 weeks and expectant vaginal delivery
D Oral aciclovir starting immediately and elective caesarean section
E Oral aciclovir starting at 36 weeks and elective caesarean section

12. A 22-year-old woman visits her GP to discuss contraceptive options. She is keen to receive effective contraception but is concerned about gaining weight. Which contraceptive has a proven association with weight gain?

A Combined oral contraceptive pill
B Progesterone only pill
C Progesterone implant
D Contraceptive injection
E Levonorgestrel intrauterine system

13. A 28-year-old woman, who is 32 weeks' pregnant, presents to the antenatal clinic after developing a widespread rash on her abdomen.

On examination, there is a confluent pruritic rash extending across most of the abdomen but sparing the umbilicus. What is the most likely diagnosis?

    A Prurigo of pregnancy
    B Polymorphic eruption of pregnancy
    C Pemphigoid gestationis
    D Striae gravidarum
    E Linea nigra

14. Which of the following is a risk factor for the development of fibroids?

    A Menopause
    B Low BMI
    C Type 2 diabetes mellitus
    D Combined oral contraceptive pill
    E Afro-Caribbean ethnicity

15. A 25-year-old woman is currently in labour at 40 weeks' gestation. She has had gestational diabetes, but her blood glucose has been well controlled since the diagnosis. As the baby's head appears in the vagina, it retracts back. This occurs several times and shoulder dystocia is suspected. The emergency button is pressed, and the patient is placed in McRoberts position, but the shoulder remains stuck. What is the next most appropriate step?

    A Change position to all fours
    B Apply suprapubic pressure
    C Perform an episiotomy
    D Perform an internal rotational manoeuvre
    E Emergency caesarean section

16. A 74-year-old woman presents to the urogynaecology clinic complaining of a dragging discomfort inside her vagina. She claims that she often 'feels something coming down'. She denies any urinary symptoms or dyspareunia. On examination, a 2nd degree uterine

prolapse is observed. After providing advice on lifestyle modification, how should this patient be managed?

A Offer advice on lifestyle modification only
B Offer topical oestrogen
C Offer pelvic floor muscle training
D Offer pelvic floor muscle training and a pessary
E Offer surgical repair

17. A 39-year-old woman has presented at 11 weeks' gestation with severe morning sickness. She is started on cyclizine, given IV fluids, and an ultrasound scan is arranged. The scan reveals lambda sign. What is this suggestive of?

A Partial molar pregnancy
B Complete molar pregnancy
C Dichorionic diamniotic twin
D Monochorionic monoamniotic twin
E Monochorionic diamniotic twin

18. A 54-year-old woman is found to have mild dyskaryosis and a negative HPV test on cervical screening. What is the most appropriate follow up for this patient?

A Repeat smear in 1 year
B Repeat smear in 3 years
C Repeat smear in 5 years
D Refer to non-urgent colposcopy
E Refer to urgent colposcopy

19. A 38-year-old woman, who is 14 weeks' pregnant, attends the family planning clinic with wishes to terminate her current pregnancy. This pregnancy was unplanned, and she is already struggling to provide for her three children after losing her job 1 month ago. She is worried about the impact another baby would have on her children. Which of the clauses of the Abortion Act applies to this case?

 A Clause A
 B Clause B
 C Clause C
 D Clause D
 E Clause E

20. A 27-year-old woman presents to her GP with a 3-day history of clear vaginal discharge. Microscopy of a high vaginal swab sample reveals clue cells. What is the most appropriate management option?

 A Doxycycline
 B Ceftriaxone
 C Ofloxacin
 D Clotrimazole
 E Metronidazole

21. A 33-year-old woman, who is on long-term treatment with warfarin for a mechanical heart valve, has attended the family planning clinic. She is intending to get pregnant and would like some advice regarding her current medication. She is on 5 mg warfarin OD and a recent INR is 2.9. What is the most appropriate advice to give her?

 A Continue on current dose of warfarin
 B Reduce dose of warfarin to 2.5 mg OD
 C Switch to rivaroxaban
 D Switch to aspirin
 E Switch to enoxaparin

22. A 22-year-old woman presents with a 3-month history of pain during sex and severe period pain. The results of her investigations are shown as follows:

Urine pregnancy test: Negative
CA125: 89 U/mL (<46)
Transvaginal ultrasound: 5 cm echogenic mass on the left ovary

What is the most likely diagnosis?

A Serous cyst
B Tubo-ovarian abscess
C Endometrioma
D Dermoid cyst
E Follicular cyst

23. Which of the following marks the end of the first stage of labour?

A Full effacement of the cervix
B Full dilatation of the cervix
C Onset of regular painful contractions
D Engagement of the foetal head
E Rupture of membranes

24. A 39-year-old woman has been experiencing crampy pelvic pain. She says that her cycle is regular, but for the past few months her periods have become heavier. On examination, her uterus feels enlarged. Transvaginal ultrasound shows two submucosal fibroids, measuring 2 cm in diameter, without distortion of the uterine cavity. She currently has two children and believes that she has completed her family. How should this patient be managed?

A Myomectomy
B Tranexamic acid
C Intrauterine system
D Ibuprofen
E Combined oral contraceptive pill

25. A 36-year-old woman, who is 24 weeks' pregnant, has felt that her baby has been moving less over the last 24 hours. She first noticed kicking at 20 weeks' gestation and usually feels it regularly throughout the day. This is the first time she has experienced a reduction in movements for a prolonged period and is becoming increasingly anxious. How should this patient be investigated?

A Arrange CTG
B Arrange CTG and ultrasound scan

    C Advise her to lie on her left side and count foetal movements for 2 hours

    D Auscultate foetal heartbeat with handheld Doppler

    E Reassure and discharge

26. A 47-year-old woman presents to her GP complaining of hot flushes that are worst at night. This has been impacting on her sleep and she finds that she often feels tired and irritable during the day. This has started to impact on her relationship with her husband. She adds that she has not been having sex frequently because she has lost the desire. She has no past medical history and her last period was 4 months ago. What is the most appropriate form of hormone replacement therapy to recommend to this patient?

    A Oestrogen only pill

    B Oestrogen only patch

    C Vaginal oestrogen cream

    D Cyclical combined pill

    E Continuous combined HRT pill

27. A 28-year-old HIV-positive woman, who is 36 weeks' pregnant, would like to discuss the measures that will be taken to reduce the risk of her child having HIV. She has been on antiretroviral therapy throughout the pregnancy and her current viral load is 42 copies/mL. Her birth plan lists a preference for a vaginal delivery. What is the most appropriate advice to give her regarding the delivery and aftercare?

    A Elective vaginal delivery with 1–2-week course of zidovudine for the baby

    B Elective caesarean section with 1–2-week course of zidovudine for the baby

    C Elective vaginal delivery with 4–6-week course of zidovudine for the baby

    D Elective caesarean section with 4–6-week course of zidovudine for the baby

E Elective caesarean section with intrapartum zidovudine infusion for the mother

28. An 18-year-old woman presents to gynaecology outpatient clinic with heavy periods. They have been heavy since her periods started at the age of 12, but they have got progressively worse and is starting to disrupt her day-to-day functioning. A bimanual examination and ultrasound scan reveal no abnormalities. What is the most appropriate management option?

   A Combined oral contraceptive pill
   B Tranexamic acid
   C Levonorgestrel intrauterine system
   D Cyclical oral progestogens
   E Copper intrauterine device

29. What is the most common cause of secondary postpartum haemorrhage?

   A Uterine atony
   B Retained products of conception
   C Perineal tear
   D Endometritis
   E Coagulopathy

30. A 30-year-old woman, who is 10 weeks' pregnant, wishes to terminate her pregnancy. She would like to avoid surgical options and would prefer to receive her treatment at home. What is the most appropriate management option for her?

   A Misoprostol only at home
   B Mifepristone only at home
   C Mifepristone and misoprostol at home
   D Mifepristone and misoprostol at clinic
   E Methotrexate at clinic

Answers

1. B

Group B *streptococcus* (GBS) is carried in the vagina and rectum in 20–40% of women in the UK. If GBS is present during labour, the bacterium may be transmitted to the neonate. A small proportion of these neonates will develop early-onset GBS (EOGBS) sepsis, which has a high mortality rate. Risk factors include preterm delivery, preterm rupture of membranes, maternal pyrexia during labour, and a previous infant with EOGBS sepsis. To prevent EOGBS infection, the following groups of patients should receive intrapartum antibiotics:

- Women in confirmed preterm labour.
- Women who are pyrexial (38°C or more) in labour.
- Women in which GBS is detected by incidental or intentional testing in the antenatal period.
- Women with GBS urinary tract infection (growth >10^5 CFU/mL) in the antenatal period.
- Women with a previous baby with early or late onset GBS disease.

If GBS is cultured from a vaginal or rectal swab during the antenatal period, immediate treatment is not recommended, but intrapartum antibiotics are indicated. Women with GBS urinary tract infection during the antenatal period require treatment both at the time of diagnosis as well as intrapartum antibiotics. There is currently no screening programme for GBS in the UK and vaginal swabs should only be taken when clinically indicated (i.e. risk factors for EOGBS disease) and this should be done at 35–37 weeks or 3–5 weeks prior to elective delivery. Vaginal cleansing is not recommended as there is no evidence that it reduces the risk of EOGBS.

2. C

The first line management for urge incontinence is lifestyle modification (e.g. reducing caffeine intake and weight loss) and bladder training for a minimum of 6 weeks. If this is unacceptable or ineffective, an anticholinergic agent (e.g. oxybutynin, tolterodine) should be trialled. If the anticholinergic medication is ineffective or not tolerated, a different agent such as mirabegron (β_3-agonist) can be offered. Since this patient does not want to trial another medication, an invasive procedure should be considered. Before these can be offered, urodynamic studies are required to better characterise the nature of the incontinence. Botulinum toxin type A injection is considered the first line invasive procedure for detrusor overactivity and is injected cytoscopically into the detrusor muscle, thereby blocking neuromuscular transmission and causing temporary paralysis. Patients need to be willing to self-catheterise as it carries the risk of causing temporary urinary retention.

Percutaneous sacral nerve stimulation is offered if an overactive bladder has not responded to botulinum toxin type A or patients are not willing to self-catheterise. It involves implanting an electrical pulse generator into the buttock which provides continuous stimulation to the S3 nerve root, thereby suppressing detrusor activity. Surgical procedures are reserved for patients with debilitating symptoms and those who have failed to respond to neuromodulation. These include augmentation cystoplasty (increasing the size of the bladder by adding tissue from the intestinal tract) and urinary diversion (redirecting the flow of urine through an opening in the abdomen, instead of into the bladder). Colposuspension is a surgical procedure used to treat stress urinary incontinence that involves elevating the bladder neck and anchoring it to Cooper's ligament.

3. E
Amniotic fluid embolism (AFE) is an obstetric emergency that occurs when foetal antigens enter the maternal circulation. It usually occurs during delivery or in the immediate postpartum period but may also occur following spontaneous or artificial rupture of membranes or during caesarean section. It is one of the main causes of maternal mortality during labour. Despite the name, AFE is not a mechanical obstruction — amniotic fluid is soluble in blood and any accompanying tissue debris will be too small to obstruct the vasculature. Instead, exposure to foetal antigens during delivery triggers an inflammatory cascade that results in organ damage and activation of the coagulation cascade, resulting in

disseminated intravascular coagulation (DIC). Risk factors for AFE include caesarean delivery, advanced maternal age, multiple pregnancy, antepartum haemorrhage, and induction of labour. AFE presents with a triad of acute hypoxia, hypotension, and coagulopathy (e.g. bleeding from uterus, surgical incisions, and venepuncture sites). Respiratory failure with cyanosis and pulmonary oedema often develops rapidly and some patients will go into cardiac arrest. The diagnosis is clinical, and management is conservative (with resuscitation, oxygen, fluids, and blood products). If it occurs during labour, immediate operative delivery is essential for the survival of the foetus, but it does not improve maternal outcomes.

Pulmonary embolism (PE) is an important differential as this patient is post-surgical and presenting with hypoxia, but PE is less likely to cause DIC and bleeding. Eclampsia is a complication of pre-eclampsia that causes seizures and may progress to coma. Uterine inversion describes a complication of the active third stage of labour where the fundus collapses into the uterine cavity. It presents with massive postpartum haemorrhage, severe abdominal pain and examination will find a uterine fundus that is not palpable abdominally. Uterine rupture is tearing of the uterus that may result in expulsion of the foetus into the abdomen. It most often occurs due to extension of a previous caesarean scar on a background of induction of labour and obstructed labour. Rupture of the uterus presents with acute onset abdominal pain, CTG abnormalities, and an abrupt termination of contractions.

4. B

This patient has the characteristic features of trichomoniasis, a common, sexually transmitted infection caused by infection with the protozoa, *Trichomonas vaginalis* (TV). Patients often report green, frothy, foul-smelling discharge with vulval itching, vaginal burning, dysuria, and pain or bleeding on sexual intercourse. The punctate haemorrhages on the cervix (also known as *strawberry cervix*) is a textbook feature of TV, however, it is relatively rare. TV is diagnosed by wet mount microscopy. This is a technique in which a sample of vaginal discharge is placed on a slide with saline and viewed under a microscope. TV is a flagellate protozoon with a characteristic 'pear' shape. TV is treated with metronidazole.

Co-infection with *Chlamydia trachomatis* and *Neisseria gonorrhoea* is common, but most patients are asymptomatic. These infectious agents can, however, spread into the reproductive organs and cause pelvic inflammatory disease. Bacterial vaginosis (BV) is the most common cause of abnormal vaginal discharge and is usually caused by an overgrowth of *Gardnerella vaginalis* and anaerobic bacteria. Patients may describe a clear, homogenous discharge which has a characteristic 'fishy' smell. It does not tend to cause vaginal burning or itching. Vulvovaginal candidiasis causes a thick, white, curd-like vaginal discharge with vaginal discomfort, dysuria, and vulval erythema.

5. B

Antenatal corticosteroids are an exceptionally important intervention in obstetrics, and they play a vital role in preventing respiratory distress in preterm infants. Surfactant is a liquid composed mainly of phospholipids which reduces the surface tension within alveoli, thereby preventing their collapse during expiration. Surfactant starts being produced by around 30 weeks' gestation and most foetuses will have an adequate amount of surfactant by around 36 weeks. Preterm infants (<37 weeks) may have an inadequate amount of surfactant to allow satisfactory lung function, therefore, when a preterm delivery is anticipated, corticosteroids are administered to the mother as it stimulates the production of surfactant by type 2 pneumocytes in the foetal lungs. This results in lower rates of infant respiratory distress syndrome. The most commonly used antenatal corticosteroid regimen is 2 doses of 12 mg IM betamethasone given 24 hours apart. The benefit of antenatal corticosteroids reaches its peak at about 24 hours after the initiation of therapy. An alternative regimen is 4 doses of 6 mg IM dexamethasone given 12 hours apart.

6. D

First line management of endometriosis is a short trial of simple analgesia (e.g. mefenamic acid) and hormonal treatment (e.g. combined oral contraceptive pill or a progestogen). If this is ineffective, not tolerated or contraindicated, surgical options should be considered.

The most appropriate surgical option depends on the importance of fertility and the location of the endometriosis. If fertility is not currently a priority (as in this case) and endometriosis does not involve the bowel, bladder or ureters, she should be offered laparoscopic excision, and this should be followed by hormonal treatment to prolong the benefits of surgery. For deep endometriosis involving the bowel, bladder or ureters, 3 months of gonadotrophin-releasing hormone agonists may be given before surgery to induce a menopausal state. Hysterectomy may also be considered if fertility is no longer required and the symptoms are severe. If fertility is a priority (i.e. the patient is currently trying to get pregnant) and endometriosis does not involve the bowel, bladder, or ureters, excision or ablation plus adhesiolysis (or laparoscopic ovarian cystectomy for endometriomas) should be offered. These treatments should not be followed by hormonal treatment as it will impair fertility. Since this patient is not actively trying to conceive, the most appropriate management is laparoscopic excision followed by hormonal treatment. Myomectomy is a fertility-sparing procedure used to treat fibroids and endometrial ablation is used to treat heavy menstrual bleeding but does not preserve fertility.

7. A

Eclamptic seizures are both prevented and treated with a magnesium sulphate infusion. A loading dose of 4 g is given over 5–10 minutes followed by an infusion of 1 g/hour. Treatment should continue until 24 hours after delivery or after the last seizure. In patients with severe pre-eclampsia and patients who have suffered eclamptic seizures, expedited delivery is vital.

Once a IV magnesium sulphate infusion is set up, it is particularly important to monitor the patient's respiratory rate, as magnesium toxicity causes respiratory depression. Magnesium sulphate toxicity can also cause arrhythmias (therefore, an ECG should be performed) and may cause loss of deep tendon reflexes. In the event of magnesium sulphate toxicity, the infusion should be stopped, and 10 mL 10% calcium gluconate should be administered over 10 minutes.

Temperature and blood pressure should be monitored periodically through labour, however, a change in temperature is not a feature of magnesium sulphate toxicity. A continuous CTG should be conducted throughout labour to monitor foetal wellbeing, however, it would not be used to identify magnesium sulphate toxicity. Low urine output is a common feature of labour in a patient with pre-eclampsia and should be monitored in case a fluid challenge is necessary.

8. B

This patient is presenting with secondary amenorrhoea and infertility on a background of extensive gynaecological surgery. Asherman syndrome is characterised by the formation of intrauterine adhesions leading to amenorrhoea due to physical obstruction of the cervix or destruction of the endometrial lining. It typically occurs in patients who have had several gynaecological operations (e.g. caesarean section, myomectomy, dilatation, and evacuation). As it causes amenorrhoea by creating a mechanical obstruction, the hormone profile will be normal. It is diagnosed by hysteroscopy, during which adhesiolysis can be performed to help relieve symptoms.

Turner syndrome is a chromosomal disorder in which females only have on X chromosome. It causes primary amenorrhoea and premature ovarian insufficiency due to hypogonadotrophic hypogonadism (which gives rise to a reduced FSH, LH, and oestradiol). Kallmann syndrome is a genetic disorder characterised by delayed or absent puberty due to a deficiency of gonadotrophin releasing hormone (hypogonadotrophic hypogonadism). Sheehan syndrome is hypopituitarism caused by ischaemic necrosis of the pituitary gland following blood loss during or after childbirth. It may cause agalactorrhoea and secondary amenorrhoea following delivery, and blood results would show a reduced FSH, LH, TSH, oestradiol, and prolactin. Polycystic ovarian syndrome causes an elevated LH and FSH with an LH:FSH ratio greater than 1:1 and the associated hyperinsulinaemia results in an elevated testosterone and reduced sex hormone binding globulin.

9. E

The second stage of labour begins when the cervix is fully dilated and ends with the birth of the baby. To understand the mechanisms of the second stage of labour, it is important to have a basic understanding of the pelvic dimensions.

	Transverse diameter	Antero-posterior diameter
Pelvic inlet	13 cm	11 cm
Pelvic outlet	11 cm	13 cm

Since the transverse diameter of the pelvic inlet is greater than the antero-posterior diameter, the widest circumference of the foetal head descends in a transverse position. The head is then encouraged to rotate as it approaches the pelvic outlet from a transverse position to an anterior–posterior position as the antero-posterior diameter of the pelvis is greater. There are nine movements that occur as the foetus passes through the birth canal:

1. **Descent:** The foetus descends into the pelvis in an occipo-trans-verse position (i.e. the foetus is facing the left or right of the mother's pelvis).
2. **Engagement:** The largest diameter of the foetal head descends into the pelvis.
3. **Flexion:** When the foetal head reaches the pelvic floor, it flexes its neck to present the smallest diameter of the foetal skull to the pelvic outlet.
4. **Internal Rotation:** The foetal head rotates 90° from an occipito-transverse position to an occipito-anterior position (i.e. the foetus is facing the mother's sacrum).
5. **Extension:** The foetal head extends and the occiput slips beneath the suprapubic arch.
6. **Crowning:** The widest part of the foetal head has negotiated the narrowest part of the pelvis. The head is visible at the vulva and does not retreat between contractions.
7. **External Rotation:** After delivery of the foetal head, it externally rotates (i.e. to face the thigh of the mother) and shoulders are in the antero-posterior plane.
8. **Delivery of the Shoulders and Body:** Downwards traction from the midwife will allow delivery of the anterior shoulder below the suprapubic arch. This is followed by upward traction to allow delivery of the posterior shoulder and rest of the body.

10. C

The FIGO staging system is used to stage endometrial cancer, based on the findings of CT, MRI, and PET scans, and lymph node biopsy. There are four stages of endometrial cancer, which are subdivided as shown in the following table.

Stage	Description of the cancer spread
I	In the uterus only
II	Connective tissue of the cervix, but not outside of the uterus
III	Beyond the uterus and cervix, but not beyond the pelvis
IV	Beyond the pelvis

Since this patient's cancer has spread beyond the uterus and cervix, but not beyond the pelvis it is Stage III. More specifically, it can be described as IIIB, as the parametrium (fibrous tissue separating the cervix from the bladder and extending between the layers of the broad ligament) is involved. Most patients will present with Stage I disease.

11. C

Genital herpes infection during pregnancy can be dangerous if acquired around the time of delivery. Neonatal herpes infection can occur if the baby comes into contact with infected secretions as they pass through the birth canal. Neonatal herpes infection can manifest in three forms based on the areas and organs affected: skin, eyes and mouth disease, disseminated herpes, and central nervous system disease (encephalitis). If primary genital herpes occurs within 6 weeks of the expected due date, oral aciclovir should be started immediately and should continue until delivery. Planned caesarean section should also be recommended to all patients to reduce the risk of transmission during delivery. All invasive procedures during labour (e.g. instrumental delivery) should be avoided.

If primary genital herpes occurs in the first or second trimester, oral aciclovir should be given from 36 weeks until delivery and an expectant vaginal delivery is possible as it is likely that the sores would have healed by the estimated due date. Herpes infection is mainly a clinical diagnosis and PCR to confirm the diagnosis provides supportive evidence but is not absolutely necessary. A recurrent episode of genital herpes during pregnancy is not an indication for caesarean section as the lesions are less likely to transmit herpes to the baby. Nonetheless, in cases of recurrent genital herpes, invasive procedures during labour should be avoided and oral aciclovir should be considered from 36 weeks' gestation.

12. D

Although there are anecdotal reports of weight gain with most forms of contraception, the only form of contraception with a proven association is the medroxyprogesterone acetate contraceptive injection (the brand, Depo-Provera, is most commonly used in the UK). The contraceptive injection is usually injected into the buttock every 12–13 weeks and it works by inhibiting ovulation. The contraceptive injection does not interrupt sex, is unaffected by other medications, and is a useful option for patients who cannot take oestrogen-based contraception. It may, however, cause irregular periods, headaches, and worsening acne. Furthermore, it can delay the return of periods by up to 1 year, so it would not be appropriate for patients who would like their fertility to return soon after stopping contraception.

13. B

Polymorphic eruption of pregnancy is a self-limiting pruritic condition that usually appears in the third trimester. It is more common in multiple pregnancies. The rash often begins in the lower abdomen involving pregnancy-associated striae and extending to the thighs, buttocks, and limbs. It tends to spare the umbilicus and the lesions often become confluent.

Prurigo of pregnancy is a common condition characterised by the presence of excoriated papules on the extensor surfaces of the limbs, abdomen, and shoulders. Pemphigoid gestationis is a rare pruritic autoimmune disorder characterised by the presence of blisters that begin on the abdomen and become widespread. Striae gravidarum are stretch marks that develop on the abdomen during pregnancy due to rapid stretching of the skin leading to tears in the dermis. They appear as reddish, purple lesions. Linea nigra is a line of hyperpigmentation that arises across the midline of the abdomen during pregnancy. It is thought to occur due to an increase in melanocyte-stimulating hormone produced by the placenta.

14. E

A fibroid (also known as leiomyoma) is a common benign tumour of the uterine smooth muscle. The tumours are oestrogen-dependent, so risk factors that increase a patient's exposure to oestrogen will increase their risk of developing fibroids, for example, early puberty and obesity. Fibroids can cause heavy menstrual bleeding, pelvic pain, and fertility issues. After menopause, fibroids typically reduce in size and symptoms tend to improve. Fibroids are particularly common in patients of Afro-Caribbean origin. There is no association between type 2 diabetes mellitus and fibroids. The levonorgestrel intrauterine system (Mirena) can be used to treat the heavy menstrual bleeding caused by fibroids.

15. B

Shoulder dystocia is an obstetric emergency in which the anterior shoulder of the foetus gets stuck behind the mother's pubic bone. It requires prompt intervention as it can lead to brachial plexus injuries, foetal hypoxia, and maternal perineal damage. Risk factors for shoulder dystocia include diabetes mellitus, maternal obesity, induced labour, and foetal macrosomia. The first step in the management of shoulder dystocia is calling for help. The patient shoulder then be placed in McRoberts manouevre (hips flexed and abducted). McRoberts manouevre is successful in most cases, however, if it fails to dislodge the anterior shoulder, suprapubic pressure should be applied. If unsuccessful, an episiotomy should be considered to create more space for manoeuvres. Then, an attempt should be made to deliver the posterior arm and shoulder or use internal rotational manoeuvres (e.g. Rubin, Woods' screw). If all the aforementioned measures are ineffective, the patient should be placed on all fours and the manoeuvres should be repeated. As a last resort, extreme measures such as a symphysiotomy (dividing the mother's pubic symphysis), cleidotomy (dividing the foetal clavicles), or the Zavenelli manoeuvres (pushing the foetal head back into the vagina in anticipation of a caesarean section) may be performed.

The step-wise management of shoulder dystocia is summarised in the following RevChart.

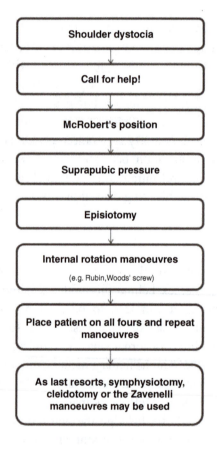

16. D

Pelvic organ prolapse is defined as protrusion of a pelvic organ beyond normal anatomical confines. The bladder, urethra, uterus, vagina, rectum, and bowel can all be involved. Prolapse occurs due to a weakened pelvic floor. Predisposing factors include childbirth, old age, obesity, long-term constipation, and heavy lifting. There are four main types of prolapse:

- **Cystocele:** Prolapse of the anterior vaginal wall, involving the bladder. This is often associated with urethral prolapse, in which it is termed cystourethrocele.
- **Uterine prolapse:** Prolapse of the uterus, cervix, and upper vagina.
- **Enterocele:** Prolapse of the upper posterior vaginal wall, involving loops of bowel.
- **Rectocele:** Prolapse of the lower posterior vaginal wall, involving the rectum.

Urogenital prolapse is classified according to the degree of severity:

- **First degree:** The lowest part of the prolapse descends halfway down the vaginal axis to the introitus.
- **Second degree:** The lowest part of the prolapse extends to the level of the introitus and protrudes through the introitus on straining.
- **Third degree:** The lowest part of the prolapse extends through the introitus and lies outside the vagina.
- **Procidentia:** Severe third degree prolapse, where the uterus lies entirely outside the vagina and is associated with complications, such as ulceration.

Women with prolapse should be advised to lose weight, minimise heavy lifting, and maintain a balanced diet high in fibre to prevent constipation. Topical oestrogen may be offered if there are signs of vaginal atrophy, such as dryness, dyspareunia, pruritus vulvae, vaginal spotting, or urinary symptoms. A 16-week course of supervised pelvic floor muscle training is advised in symptomatic pelvic organ prolapse and this is often in conjunction with a vaginal pessary. These are rubber or silicone devices that are inserted into the vagina to support the pelvic organs. Pessaries are changed every 6 months and may be given with topical oestrogen to reduce the risk of vaginal erosion. Other possible complications include bacterial vaginosis, urinary tract infections, stress incontinence, and interference with intercourse. Surgical management is offered to women whose symptoms have not improved with conservative measures. The patient in this case has a symptomatic prolapse without vaginal atrophy, so pelvic floor training in combination with a pessary is most appropriate.

17. C

Multiple pregnancies are typically first identified at the dating scan. Multiple pregnancies are associated with a number of antenatal complications including hyperemesis gravidarum (described in this SBA). The dating scan aims, not only to date the pregnancy, but to determine its chorionicity as this affects ongoing management. Twin pregnancies can be dichorionic diamniotic (2 placentas, 2 amniotic sacs), monochorionic monoamniotic (1 placenta, 1 amniotic sac) or monochorionic diamniotic (1 placenta, 2 amniotic sacs) based on the time at which a zygote divides before implantation. Dichorionic diamniotic twins may arise from 2 separate zygotes or due to 1 zygote dividing within 3 days of fertilisation. Monochorionic diamniotic twins arise when the zygote divides between day 4 and 8 after fertilisation. Monochorionic monoamniotic twins arise when the zygote divides more than 8 days after fertilisation.

Lambda sign is an ultrasound feature of dichorionic pregnancies where the gap between the two amniotic membranes forms a wedge shape. It is also sometimes referred to as twin peak sign. T-sign is when the junction between the intertwin membrane and the placenta forms a right angle, and it is suggestive of a monochorionic diamniotic pregnancy. In monochorionic monoamniotic twins, there will be no intertwin membrane. Molar pregnancy can cause hyperemesis gravidarum and a large-for-dates uterus, however, it typically has a characteristic 'snowstorm' or 'bunch of grapes' appearance on ultrasound.

18. C

The NHS cervical screening programme is offered every 3 years for women between the ages of 25 and 50, and every 5 years for women between the ages of 50 and 64. Cervical screening uses liquid-based cytology to look for the presence of dyskaryosis (abnormal nuclear morphology) and to test for human papilloma virus (HPV). Dyskaryosis is classified according to degree of severity into borderline, mild, moderate, and severe. Dyskaryosis is not the same as cervical intraepithelial neoplasia (CIN), which is a histological diagnosis made after colposcopy and biopsy. The results of the cervical smear determine the follow-up necessary, as illustrated in the following table.

Abnormality	Management
Normal	Repeat smear in 3 or 5 years depending on patient's age
Inflammatory	Repeat in 6 months and refer to colposcopy if three consecutive abnormal smears
Borderline nuclear changes	High risk HPV test: Refer for non-urgent colposcopy (within 6 weeks) if positive, repeat smear in 3 or 5 years if negative
Mild dyskaryosis	High risk HPV test: Refer to non-urgent colposcopy if positive, repeat smear in 3 or 5 years if negative
Moderate dyskaryosis	Refer to urgent colposcopy (within 2 weeks)
Severe dyskaryosis	Refer to urgent colposcopy (within 2 weeks)
Invasion suspected	Refer to urgent colposcopy (within 2 weeks)
Abnormal glandular cells	Refer to colposcopy
Three inadequate samples in a row	Refer to non-urgent colposcopy
HIV positive patient	Smear test annually

This patient's smear shows mild dyskaryosis with a negative HPV test. She does therefore not require colposcopy and can return to the routine cervical screening programme. Since this patient is above the age of 50 years, her next smear will be in 5 years.

19. D

The Abortion Act 1967 outlines the conditions under which a termination of pregnancy can be conducted. The clauses are listed as follows.

Clause	Grounds
A	Continuance of the pregnancy would involve risk to the life of the pregnant woman greater than if the pregnancy were terminated.
B	Termination is necessary to prevent grave or permanent injury to the physical or mental health of the woman.
C	Pregnancy has not exceeded its 24th week and continuance would involve a greater risk of injury to the physical or mental health of the woman than if it was terminated.
D	Pregnancy has not exceeded its 24th week and continuance would involve greater risk of injury, than if the pregnancy were terminated, to the physical or mental health of any existing children of the family of the pregnant woman.
E	There is substantial risk that if the child were born, it would suffer from such physical or mental abnormalities as to be significantly handicapped.
F	Termination is needed to save the life of the pregnant woman.
G	Termination is needed to prevent grave permanent injury to the physical and mental health of the pregnant woman.

20. E

Bacterial vaginosis (BV) is a disease affecting the vagina caused by an imbalance in the normal vaginal flora. The most common presenting symptom is a new white or grey vaginal discharge which has a characteristic 'fishy' odour. It is, however, worth noting that many women with BV will not have any symptoms. BV can be diagnosed using the Amsel criteria:

- Thin, white, homogenous vaginal discharge
- Clue cells on microscopy
- pH of vaginal fluid >4.5
- Fishy odour when potassium hydroxide is added to vaginal fluid

The presence of three out of the four criteria is diagnostic of BV.

BV is treated with a 5–7 day course of metronidazole. Topical clinda-mycin is an alternative that can be used in metronidazole and is not tolerated. Patients should also be advised to avoid excessive genital washing or vaginal douching. It is particularly important to treat BV promptly in pregnancy as it is associated with preterm labour and chorioamnionitis.

In the context of genitourinary medicine, doxycycline is used to treat chlamydia, ceftriaxone is used for gonorrhoea, ofloxacin is used as an alternative treatment for pelvic inflammatory disease, and clotrimazole is used for vulvovaginal candidiasis. A combination of ceftriaxone, doxycycline, and metronidazole is used as the first-line treatment for pelvic inflammatory disease.

21. E

Warfarin is contraindicated in the first trimester as it is associated with birth defects, stillbirth, and neonatal death. This can be difficult to manage in patients who require warfarin for a critical indication, such as prevention of stroke in patients with mechanical valves. Patients requiring anticoagulation during pregnancy should instead be switched to a low molecular weight heparin (e.g. enoxaparin), ideally before conception.

Rivaroxaban is a direct oral anticoagulant (DOAC) which is a class of orally-active anticoagulant that has become more prominent in medical practice over the past few decades. It is a direct factor Xa inhibitor, thereby inhibiting the intrinsic and extrinsic pathways of the clotting cascade. Although there is little evidence in humans, it is recommended that DOACs are avoided in pregnancy as they have been shown to be embryotoxic in animal studies. Other examples of DOACs include dabigatran and apixaban. Aspirin is an antiplatelet (not an anticoagulant) so it is effective at preventing platelet activation and clumping in response to vessel wall injury, however, it is not effective on its own to prevent clot formation in patients with mechanical heart valves.

22. C

An endometrioma is a type of ovarian cyst that is formed by endometrial tissue. It causes deep dyspareunia and dysmenorrhoea, and has a characteristic echogenic 'ground glass' appearance on transvaginal ultrasound scan. It can also cause issues with fertility. CA125 is a tumour marker for ovarian cancer that is also often raised in cases of endometrioma.

Benign ovarian cysts can be categorised based on their origin. Functional cysts are the most common type of cyst and can either form from follicles (follicular cysts) or from the corpus luteum (corpus luteal cysts). As follicles are a normal physiological phenomenon, they are only considered cysts once the diameter exceeds 3 cm. Theca lutein cysts are a type of bilateral functional cyst that occur due to excessive stimulation by β-hCG. As a result, they are associated with gestational trophoblastic disease and multiple pregnancies. Germ cell tumours mainly refer to dermoid cysts (also known as mature teratomas) which are the most common type of cyst in young women. They contain fully differentiated tissue types from all three germ cell layers. They tend to be large and can lead to ovarian torsion. Epithelial cysts are most common in perimenopausal women and there are three main types: serous, mucinous, and Brenner tumours. Sex cord stromal tumours arise from the stromal component of the ovary — they also have three main types: fibroma, thecoma, and granulosa cell tumour.

23. B

Labour is divided into three main stages with clear start and end points summarised in the following table.

Stage	Phase	Start point	End point	Normal duration
1st Stage	Latent	Onset of regular, painful contractions	3–4 cm dilatation of the cervix	3–8 hours
	Active	End of latent phase	Full dilatation (10 cm) of the cervix	2–6 hours
2nd Stage	Passive	End of 1st stage	Onset of involuntary expulsive contractions	1–2 hours
	Active	Onset of maternal urge to push	Delivery of the baby	<2 hours
3rd Stage		End of 2nd stage	Delivery of placenta and membranes	<30 mins

24. C

Fibroids (leiomyomas) are benign tumours consisting of smooth muscle cells and fibroblasts that develop in women of reproductive age. They may develop anywhere within the myometrium and are described as either: subserosal, intramural, or submucosal. Subserosal fibroids are on the outer surface of the uterus so may cause pressure symptoms on surrounding structures (e.g. urinary symptoms from pressure on the bladder). On the other hand, intramural and submucosal fibroids are more likely to cause gynaecological issues such as heavy menstrual bleeding and subfertility.

Treatment is not necessary for asymptomatic fibroids as they shrink following the menopause. If fibroids are symptomatic, less than 3 cm and not distorting the uterine cavity, first-line management is the levonorgestrel intrauterine system (IUS) which helps relieve the heavy menstrual bleeding. If the IUS is not suitable, other hormonal contraceptives, such as the combined oral contraceptive pill and progesterone only pill, can be used. If hormonal treatment is unacceptable or the patient is trying to get pregnant, tranexamic acid (anti-fibrinolytic) and non-steroidal anti-inflammatory agents (such as mefenamic acid or ibuprofen) should be recommended. Since this patient has a small symptomatic fibroid without uterine distortion and no desire to conceive, the IUS is the most appropriate management option. Myomectomy is a surgical procedure that removed fibroids from the uterine wall. It is an effective treatment for fibroids but is not considered the first-line treatment option.

25. D

Most women become aware of foetal movements from 18–20 weeks' gestation but foetal activity may be felt as early as 16 weeks' gestation in multiparous women. The frequency of movements tends to increase until around 32 weeks' gestation, and then plateaus until the onset of labour. There is no generic normal range for foetal movements — pregnant women are instead advised to report any changes in the patterns that they are used to. Foetal movements show diurnal variation and movements are usually absent during foetal sleep cycles that occur regularly throughout the day and night, and usually last 20–40 minutes. After 28 weeks' gestation, if women are unsure if movements are reduced, they should be advised to lie on their left side and count foetal movements for 2 hours. If they do not feel at least 10, they should contact their maternity unit immediately. Investigation is essential as reduced foetal movements may be a sign of foetal distress.

When a woman presents with reduced foetal movements, the first step is to determine foetal viability using a handheld Doppler to confirm the presence of a foetal heartbeat. If foetal viability has been confirmed and the pregnancy is over 28 weeks' gestation, a CTG is indicated. Ultrasound scan is also required after 28 weeks' gestation if reduced foetal movements persist despite a normal CTG or if there are any additional risk factors for stillbirth or foetal growth restriction. Women can be reassured that 70% of pregnancies with a single episode of reduced foetal movements are uncomplicated and should be advised to return if they have a second episode. Since this patient is less than 28 weeks' pregnant, foetal viability should be confirmed with a handheld Doppler.

26. D

The menopause occurs at an average age of 51, however, it can occur at any age above 40 years. The typical symptoms of the menopause include hot flushes, night sweats, reduced libido, vaginal dryness, and mood changes. The symptoms are thought to arise due to reducing levels of oestrogen. Hormone replacement therapy (HRT) provides supplementary oestrogen thereby blunting the symptoms experienced. HRT can be delivered in a number of different preparations depending on numerous patient factors. In most women, oestrogen must be given with a progestogen component to counteract the stimulatory effect of oestrogen on the endometrium, thereby reducing the risk of developing endometrial cancer. In women without a uterus (i.e. post-hysterectomy), oestrogen-only preparations can be safely used. Women who are predominantly suffering from vaginal symptoms may be treated with vaginal oestrogen cream, which can reduce dryness and aid sexual functioning but does not have systemic effects.

Combined HRT can be given continuously (an oestrogen and progestogen every day) or cyclically (an oestrogen every day for 1–3 months and a progestogen for the last 14 days to precipitate a withdrawal bleed). A continuous regimen is preferred for women who are post-menopausal (i.e.

have not had a period for over 1 year) whereas a cyclical regime is preferred for women who are peri-menopausal (i.e. have not had a period for less than 1 year). As the patient in this question is peri-menopausal and has a uterus, a cyclical combined pill would be the best option.

27. C

The management of HIV in pregnancy focuses on reducing the risk of vertical transmission to the unborn child. All patients should commence or continue antiretroviral therapy throughout the pregnancy. Patients should also be monitored closely by measuring viral load every 2–4 weeks, at 36 weeks, and after delivery. Planned vaginal delivery is possible in patients who have a viral load less than 50 copies/mL at 36 weeks' gestation. If the viral load is higher or the patient has a hepatitis C coinfection, planned caesarean section is recommended. Women with a high viral load should also receive IV zidovudine if undergoing a planned caesarean section or if they present with spontaneous rupture of membranes. All babies born to mothers who are HIV-positive should receive a 4–6 week course of oral antiretroviral therapy (usually zidovudine) starting within 4 hours of birth. In developed countries, it is also recommended that women avoid breastfeeding due to the risk of transmission in breastmilk. The baby should also be tested for HIV by PCR at birth, on discharge and at 6 and 12 weeks after birth. It is important to note that HIV antibody tests are likely to be positive in most babies born to HIV-positive mothers, irrespective of their own infection status, due to the passive transfer of antibodies from the mother.

28. C

Heavy menstrual bleeding (HMB) is a common gynaecological complaint that can have a serious impact on a patient's life. There are many causes of HMB including fibroids, adenomyosis, pelvic inflammatory disease, and polyps, however, often there is no identifiable cause. All patients with HMB should have a full blood count to check for anaemia. A coagulation screen should also be considered in patients with HMB since menarche. Other investigations for an underlying cause include ultrasound scans, swabs, and hysteroscopy.

Decisions on managing HMB is dependent on a number of factors, most importantly, the patient's intentions on getting pregnant and need for contraception. In patients who are not intending to get pregnant, a levonorgestrel intrauterine system is the first-line treatment option. Second-line hormonal options include the combined oral contraceptive pill and cyclical oral progestogens. In patients who are trying to get pregnant or would like to avoid hormonal treatments, tranexamic acid can help reduce the bleeding without reducing the chances of getting pregnant. In patients who have completed their families, surgical options such as endometrial ablation and hysterectomy may be considered. The copper intrauterine device often makes periods heavier and more painful in the weeks or months after insertion.

The management of HMB is summarised in the following RevChart.

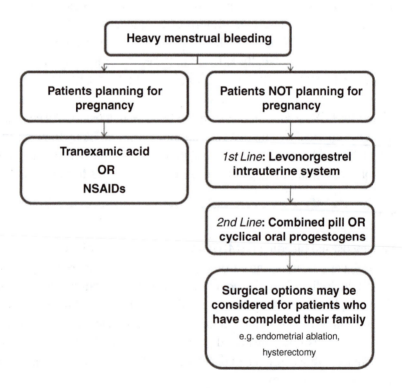

29. D

A secondary postpartum haemorrhage (PPH) is defined as blood loss in excess of 500 mL occurring between 24 hours and 12 weeks after delivery. The most common cause of secondary PPH is uterine infection (endometritis). Patients are likely to have a fever and be generally unwell along with vaginal bleeding. It usually requires admission to hospital for IV antibiotics. Other causes of secondary PPH include retained products of conception, local trauma (e.g. perineal tears), and coagulopathy. Uterine atony is the most common cause of primary PPH (haemorrhage that occurs within 24 hours of delivery).

30. D

Medical termination of pregnancy consists of administering oral mifepristone followed 24–48 hours later by misoprostol (vaginal, buccal, or sublingual). Mifepristone is a selective progesterone receptor modulator which promotes the breakdown of the endometrium. Misoprostol is a prostaglandin E_2 analogue which promotes cervical ripening and uterine contractions, thereby facilitating the expulsion of the pregnancy tissue. Medical termination is theoretically possible at any gestation, however, it is more successful at earlier gestations as larger foetal parts are more difficult to pass. The guidelines recommend that terminations of pregnancies of 12 or more weeks' gestation should be conducted in a clinical setting due to an increased risk of bleeding and because repeated doses of misoprostol may be needed. Terminations at earlier gestations can be conducted at home provided the patient can be followed up easily. Patients should be informed that the bleeding can continue for 2 weeks, and a pregnancy test should be performed after 3 weeks. If a medical termination is performed after 21^{+6} weeks, an intracardiac potassium chloride injection should be administered to the foetus to eliminate the possibility of the aborted foetus showing any signs of life.

Misoprostol alone is used to treat miscarriages. Methotrexate is the medical treatment of choice for ectopic pregnancies.

Obstetrics and Gynaecology: Paper 4

Questions

1. A 32-year-old woman has been struggling to get pregnant for the last 15 months. She has always had irregular periods which were temporarily controlled by the combined oral contraceptive pill which has been discontinued since she started trying to get pregnant. She has a BMI of 24 kg/m² and a transvaginal ultrasound scan reveals 22 cysts on both ovaries. What is the best management option to improve her chances of getting pregnant?

    A Recommend weight loss
    B Clomiphene citrate
    C Refer for *in vitro* fertilisation
    D Metformin
    E Laparoscopic ovarian drilling

2. A 22-year-old woman, who is 8 weeks' pregnant, presents to her booking appointment. When discussing vaccination history, she explains that she did not have the MMR vaccine as a child. She is concerned about the risks of developing an infection during her pregnancy. Serology confirms that she has no immunity against measles, mumps, or rubella. What is the most appropriate management option?

    A Offer MMR vaccination at next antenatal appointment
    B Offer MMR vaccination after pregnancy is complete
    C Offer rubella vaccine only
    D 2-weekly ultrasound scans
    E 4-weekly ultrasound scans

3. A 38-year-old woman attends the colposcopy clinic after a routine smear reveals moderate dyskaryosis. A punch biopsy of the transformation zone is taken. Histological analysis reveals dyskaryotic cells in the lower third of the cervical epithelium. What is the most appropriate management option?

    A Large loop excision of the transformation zone
    B Cone biopsy
    C Repeat smear in 6 months
    D Repeat smear in 12 months
    E Return to routine recall

4. A 25-year-old woman has just given birth to a baby boy at 37 weeks' gestation. She required a forceps delivery due to failure to progress in the second stage. She has sustained a tear to her perineal muscle without involvement of the anal sphincter. Which degree of perineal tear is this?

    A 1st degree
    B 2nd degree
    C 3a degree
    D 3b degree
    E 4th degree

5. A 69-year-old woman presents to the urogynaecology clinic complaining that she often feels a lump coming out of her vagina. She sometimes has to rush to the toilet and at other times she is unable to pass any urine at all. On examination, a 3rd degree cystourethrocele is identified. The patient is unhappy with the results of her pelvic floor training programme and is unable to tolerate a pessary. She

wants to discuss surgical options. What is the most appropriate management option for this patient?

A Vaginal sacrospinous fixation
B Sacrocolpopexy
C Vaginal sacrospinous hysteropexy
D Posterior repair
E Anterior repair

6. A 35-year-old woman with known pre-eclampsia, who is 34 weeks' pregnant, is admitted to the antenatal ward after experiencing severe epigastric pain and some visual changes. On examination, her symphysis fundal height is 30 cm, the foetus has a transverse lie and the foetal heart rate is 156 bpm. Her blood pressure is 178/112 mm Hg but her other vital signs are normal. Her blood results are shown as follows:

Hb: 98 g/L (115–160)
MCV: 104 fL (82–100)
Platelets: 65×10^9/L (150–400)
WCC: 11.4×10^9/L (4–11)
CRP: 2 mg/L (<3)
ALT: 568 iU/L (3–40)
AST: 870 iU/L (3–30)
ALP: 204 µmol/L (33–96)
GGT: 16 iU/L (9–58)
Bilirubin: 32 µmol/L (3–17)

What is the most likely diagnosis?

A Biliary colic
B Cholecystitis
C HELLP syndrome
D Obstetric cholestasis
E Acute fatty liver of pregnancy

7. A 19-year-old woman presents to the GP for advice on contraception. After discussing her options and making a decision, the GP warns her that this particular type of contraception may cause heavier, longer and more painful periods. Which method of contraception has she chosen?

    A Levonorgestrel intrauterine system
    B Copper intrauterine device
    C Contraceptive implant
    D Progesterone-only pill
    E Contraceptive injection

8. A 26-year-old woman with epilepsy attends the family planning clinic as she would like to start a family and wants to find out more about the impact of her epilepsy on a future pregnancy. She is currently on lamotrigine to prevent seizures. She has had four tonic clonic seizures in the past 12 months. What is the most appropriate management option?

    A Discontinue treatment and start 400 μg folic acid
    B Discontinue treatment and start 5 mg folic acid
    C Continue treatment and start 2.5 mg folic acid
    D Continue treatment and start 5 mg folic acid
    E Change to valproate and start 5 mg folic acid

9. A 72-year-old woman has developed some vaginal itchiness. For the last 6 months, she has noticed some white patches surrounding her vagina and anus which are very itchy and sore. On examination, there is a white, thickened rash involving the labia, clitoral hood, and perianal skin. There is no vaginal discharge, dysuria, or involvement of the vaginal mucosa. What is the most likely diagnosis?

    A Vulval intraepithelial neoplasia
    B Vulval squamous cell carcinoma
    C Lichen sclerosis
    D Candidiasis
    E Atrophic vulvovaginitis

10. A 29-year-old woman has been diagnosed with a low-lying placenta following her 20-week anomaly scan. Her first child was delivered by emergency caesarean section due to foetal distress. She would like to know how her current condition will be managed. What is the most appropriate advice to give her?

    A Administer antenatal corticosteroids and plan elective caesarean section
    B 2-weekly CTG and ultrasound scans
    C 4-weekly CTG and ultrasound scans
    D Rescan at 28 weeks
    E Rescan at 32 weeks

11. A 41-year-old woman is being treated for a 5 cm intramural fibroid with a levonorgestrel intrauterine system and tranexamic acid. Despite this, she is still experiencing heavy periods. On examination, the uterus feels enlarged and distorted. She has not yet completed her family and wants to discuss definitive treatment options. What is the most appropriate next step in this patient's management?

    A Hysterectomy
    B Endometrial ablation
    C Goserelin acetate plus myomectomy
    D Goserelin acetate only
    E Hysteroscopic resection

12. Which of the following is a major indication for treatment with 150 mg aspirin from 12 weeks' gestation to prevent pre-eclampsia?

    A Systemic lupus erythematosus
    B Congestive cardiac failure
    C Previous gestational diabetes
    D Multiple pregnancy
    E Family history of pre-eclampsia

13. A 38-year-old woman is being investigated for issues regarding fertility. She has never been pregnant before despite having regular unprotected sex for 3 years. She mentions that her periods have been irregular for the past 9 months. Her blood test results are shown as follows:

FSH: 40 U/L (1.2–9 U/L)
LH: 35 U/L (<14.7 U/L)
TSH: 3.5 mU/L (0–5.7 mU/L)
Prolactin: 100 IU/L (53–360 U/L)
Sex hormone binding globulin: 50 nmol/L (26–110 nmol/L)
Oestradiol: 90 pmol/L (101–905 pmol/L)
Testosterone: 1.5 nmol/L (0.2–2.9 nmol/L)
Midluteal progesterone: 15 nmol/L (>35 nmol/L)

What is the most likely diagnosis?

    A Polycystic ovarian syndrome
    B Hypogonadotrophic hypogonadism
    C Premature ovarian insufficiency
    D Hyperprolactinaemia
    E Hypothyroidism

14. A 33-year-old woman, who is 34 weeks pregnant, is referred for an ultrasound scan after her symphysis-fundal height was lower than expected for her gestation. The ultrasound reveals an abdominal circumference that has fallen from the 45th to the 19th centile. Head circumference has remained on the 40th centile. The estimated foetal weight is on the 20th centile. What is the most likely diagnosis?

    A Symmetrical growth restriction
    B Asymmetrical growth restriction
    C Small for gestational age
    D Normal finding for gestation
    E Hydrocephalus

15. A 27-year-old woman presents to A&E with left iliac fossa pain and a positive pregnancy test. A transvaginal ultrasound shows a left adnexal mass with a diameter of 40 mm. A foetal heart beat is detected. Her blood pressure is 125/90 mmHg and her heart rate is 86 bpm. On examination, there is some tenderness in the left iliac fossa and cervical motion tenderness on vaginal examination. She explains that she recently had a laparoscopy to investigate pelvic pain which incidentally found that her right fallopian tube is damaged. Her serum β-hCG is 2000 IU/L. How should this patient be managed?

    A Follow up β-hCG in 48 hours
    B Methotrexate injection
    C Urgent laparotomy
    D Laparoscopy and salpingotomy
    E Laparoscopy and salpingectomy

16. Which of the following is an expected physiological change in pregnancy?

    A Increase in tidal volume
    B Increase in protein S
    C Decrease in mean corpuscular volume
    D Decrease in platelet size
    E Decrease in glomerular filtration rate

17. A 34-year-old woman, who is 38 weeks' pregnant, would like to arrange her contraception in advance of delivering her baby. She has previously been on the levonorgestrel intrauterine system (LNG-IUS) but would consider other options if necessary. She is intending to breastfeed her baby. Which of the following is true regarding postpartum contraception?

    A No contraception is needed for 4 weeks after delivery
    B Combined oral contraceptive pill can be started after day 21
    C Contraceptive implant can only be inserted after day 21

D Breastfeeding provides effective contraception for 1 year after delivery

E LNG-IUS can be inserted within 2 days of delivery

18. A 27-year-old woman has had an induction of labour at 39 weeks' gestation. Intravaginal prostaglandin gel was last inserted 2 hours ago. Her cervix is 5 cm dilated and moderately effaced. A CTG reveals 6 contractions in 10 minutes with combined decelerations and a foetal heart rate of 112 bpm. What is the most appropriate management option?

    A Administer second dose of intravaginal prostaglandin

    B Prepare for instrumental delivery

    C Commence syntocinon infusion

    D Administer terbutaline

    E Emergency caesarean section

19. Which of the following complications is most strongly associated with polycystic ovarian syndrome?

    A Breast cancer

    B Endometrial cancer

    C Ovarian cancer

    D Type 1 diabetes mellitus

    E Central sleep apnoea

20. A 29-year-old woman, who is 35 weeks' pregnant, presents with a 2-week history of excruciating pelvic pain which sometimes spreads down her thighs. This has left her bedbound as she finds that walking is particularly painful. She occasionally hears a clicking sound when she climbs the stairs. What is the most likely diagnosis?

    A Pelvic girdle pain

    B Sciatica

    C Braxton Hicks contractions

    D Sacroiliitis

    E Spinal disc prolapse

21. A 25-year-old woman presents to the gynaecology emergency room with lower abdominal pain and offensive vaginal discharge. She has also experienced some discomfort when having sex over the last 2 months. A bimanual examination elicits cervical excitation. The results of her blood tests are shown in the following:

Hb: 121 g/L (115–160)
MCV: 86 fL (82–100)
Platelets: 212 × 10⁹/L (150–400)
WBC: 14.1 × 10⁹/L (4–11)
Neutrophils: 11.6 × 10⁹/L (2–7)
Lymphocytes: 2.4 × 10⁹/L (1–3)
CRP: 46 mg/L (<10)

Given the most likely diagnosis, which of the following is this patient most at risk of in the future?

    A Miscarriage
    B Ectopic pregnancy
    C Molar pregnancy
    D Utero-vaginal fistula
    E Chorioamnionitis

22. A 42-year-old woman is referred to foetal medicine for amniocentesis after receiving a high-risk result in the combined test for Down syndrome. She is rhesus negative and due to undergo an amniocentesis at 18 weeks' gestation. Which of the following should be included in her management?

    A 250 IU anti-D immunoglobulin only
    B 250 IU anti-D immunoglobulin and a Kleihauer test
    C 500 IU anti-D immunoglobulin only
    D 500 IU anti-D immunoglobulin and a Kleihauer test
    E 1500 IU anti-D immunoglobulin only

23. A 21-year-old woman presents with headaches and breast tenderness. The symptoms start 1 week before her period and resolve once her

period starts. She complains that, during this time, her acne worsens, and she begins to feel anxious and low. The symptoms often stop her from going to work as a beautician and she frequently cancels plans with friends. What is the most appropriate management option?

A Offer lifestyle advice only
B Offer lifestyle advice and prescribe a continuous combined oral contraceptive pill
C Offer lifestyle advice, prescribe a continuous combined oral contraceptive pill and refer for cognitive behavioural therapy
D Offer lifestyle advice, prescribe a cyclical combined oral contraceptive pill and refer for cognitive behavioural therapy
E Offer lifestyle advice, prescribe a selective serotonin reuptake inhibitor and refer for cognitive behavioural therapy

24. A 32-year-old woman, who is 32 weeks' pregnant, presents with a sudden gush of clear fluid from her vagina. A sterile speculum examination reveals pooling of liquor. She has not experienced any contractions. Her observations and CTG results are shown in the following:

Temperature: 37.1°C
Blood pressure: 110/82 mm Hg
Heart rate: 86 bpm
Respiratory rate: 12 breaths/min
CTG: met criteria within 15 minutes

What of the following would be part of her initial management?

A Emergency C-section
B Discharge and recommend awaiting the onset of contractions
C Urgently administer IV magnesium sulphate
D Begin oral erythromycin
E Begin oral nifedipine

25. A 29-year-old woman, who is 9 weeks' pregnant, presents to the gynaecology emergency room with a 5-day history of irregular, light vaginal bleeding. She has had severe morning sickness for the past

3 weeks and has recently had her booking visit. A urine pregnancy test is positive, and a bimanual examination reveals a 15-week uterus. What is the most likely diagnosis?

A Missed miscarriage
B Threatened miscarriage
C Molar pregnancy
D Ectopic pregnancy
E Fibroid red degeneration

26. A 27-year-old woman with hypothyroidism attends a family planning clinic expressing wishes to get pregnant. She is currently taking 50 µg levothyroxine daily. Thyroid function tests are requested and the results are shown as follows:

TSH: 4.1 mU/L (0.5–5.5)
Free T4: 16 pmol/L (9–18)

What is the most appropriate advice to give her?

A Stop levothyroxine and check TFTs in 2 weeks
B Remain on current dose and check TFTs in 2 weeks
C Reduce levothyroxine by 25 µg
D Reduce levothyroxine by 50 µg
E Increase levothyroxine by 25 µg

27. A 40-year-old woman, who presented with post-coital and intermenstrual bleeding, is diagnosed with cervical cancer. The tumour is confined to the cervix and is less than 4 cm in size. She has completed her family. What is the most appropriate management option for this patient?

A Conservative management
B Radical hysterectomy with lymphadenectomy
C Radical trachelectomy with lymphadenectomy
D Chemotherapy and radiotherapy
E Palliative care

28. A 35-year-old woman would like to discuss her birth plan. She has been pregnant once before, which resulted in an emergency caesarean section due to a pathological CTG trace. She found the recovery from the caesarean section difficult and would like to have a planned vaginal delivery for her current pregnancy. Which of the following is a contraindication for vaginal birth after caesarean section?

   A Singleton pregnancy
   B More than 39 weeks' gestation
   C Previous placenta praevia
   D Previous classical caesarean section
   E Cephalic presentation

29. A 20-year-old woman presents to the gynaecology emergency room with right-sided lower abdominal pain. It began suddenly whilst she was playing a hockey match. On direct questioning, she mentions that she has had some pain whilst having sex over the past 2 months but reports no abnormal vaginal bleeding. A pregnancy test is negative, and a transvaginal ultrasound reveals free fluid around her right ovary. What is the most appropriate management option?

   A Emergency laparoscopy
   B Admit for observation and analgesia
   C Admit for IV antibiotics
   D Discharge with paracetamol
   E Request serum β-hCG

30. A 37-year-old woman is currently 15 weeks' pregnant with a baby boy. She also has twin girls who are 3 years old. She has had one miscarriage at 14 weeks, a medication termination of pregnancy at 12 weeks and one stillbirth at 26 weeks. What is her gravidity and parity?

   A G5 P1
   B G5 P2
   C G5 P3
   D G6 P2
   E G6 P3

Answers

1. B

The history of irregular periods controlled by the combined oral contraceptive pill (COCP), fertility issues, and presence of multiple cysts on her ovaries are suggestive of polycystic ovarian syndrome (PCOS). The abnormal hormone levels and cyclical changes in PCOS leads to oligoovulation or anovulation resulting in difficulty getting pregnant. This patient has been trying to get pregnant for more than 12 months and a cause for her subfertility has been identified so treatment can be initiated at this stage. As this patient has a BMI within the normal range, further weight loss should not be recommended. The best treatment option would be clomiphene citrate, a selective oestrogen receptor modulator which can stimulate ovulation. This can be given with or without metformin. Clomiphene citrate is usually used for up to 6 months and is associated with an increased risk of multiple pregnancy. If clomiphene citrate is unsuccessful, a surgical procedure called laparoscopic ovarian drilling may be considered. This involves breaking down parts of the ovarian stroma with the hope that it will help induce ovulation. Patients who continue to have fertility issues despite these treatments may be considered for *in vitro* fertilisation.

Patients with PCOS who are not trying to get pregnant can regain control of their periods by using the COCP. In particular, the co-cyprindiol oral contraceptive pill may be useful in PCOS complicated by acne and hirsutism as it has anti-androgenic activity. Topical eflornithine cream is also useful for hirsutism resulting from PCOS. Recommending dietary modification and regular exercise can also help reduce the risk of developing type 2 diabetes mellitus and cardiovascular disease.

2. B

The Measles, Mumps, and Rubella (MMR) vaccine has been part of the UK childhood vaccination schedule since 1988, however, there was a decrease in the uptake of the vaccine in the late 1990s and early 2000s as a result of a fraudulent publication linking the MMR vaccine with autism.

Patients used to be screened for rubella immunity as part of routine antenatal screening, however, the low rates of rubella in the UK achieved by the vaccination programme led to removal of antenatal rubella screening in 2016. Of the three infections, rubella is most concerning in pregnancy. It can result in congenital rubella syndrome, which is characterised by cataracts, sensorineural deafness, and congenital cardiac defects (most commonly patent ductus arteriosus). Measles, although it does not cause any congenital defects, is associated with an increased risk of miscarriage, prematurity, and low birth weight. There is some evidence to suggest a link between mumps and prematurity, however, this remains inconclusive. Mumps can, however, cause orchitis and infertility in boys.

Women attending a family planning clinic before becoming pregnant should be offered the MMR vaccine as soon as possible. They should then be advised to avoid getting pregnant for 1 month after receiving the vaccine. Women who are already pregnant should not be offered the MMR vaccine during pregnancy as it is a live vaccine and carries a theoretical risk of causing a rubella infection. Therefore, the MMR vaccine should be offered after delivery. It is typically given as two doses — the first, as soon as the baby is born and the second, 4 weeks later. The rubella only vaccine is no longer available in the UK.

3. D

Cervical intraepithelial neoplasia is an abnormal change in the surface of the cervix that can progress to become cancer if left untreated. It is a histological diagnosis and has three degrees of severity depending on the portion of the epithelium that contains dysplastic cells (e.g. in CIN1, dysplastic cells are present within the lower 1/3 of the epithelium). CIN1, the mildest form of CIN, is a relatively common change which is likely to resolve spontaneously in most women. Therefore, patients should be offered a repeat smear in 12 months to check for resolution.

Patients with CIN2, CIN3, and CGIN (cervical glandular intraepithelial neoplasia) should be offered removal — usually by large loop excision of the transformation zone (LLETZ). LLETZ is a minor surgical procedure which can be performed during colposcopy and involves removing the abnormal cells using an electrically heated wire. Although it is an effective treatment for CIN, it is associated with an increased risk of miscarriage and preterm delivery due to cervical incompetence. A cone biopsy is another approach to removing abnormal cervical tissue but is performed less frequently and is used when a larger area of tissue requires removal. Patients who have undergone treatment for CIN should receive a test of cure smear 6 months later. If the punch biopsy taken during colposcopy was normal, patients can return to routine recall.

4. B

Perineal tears are a common complication of vaginal delivery, especially when instruments, such as forceps, are used. They can be graded based on the extent to which the perineum and anal sphincter complex are affected:

- **1st degree:** Superficial damage with no muscle involvement.
- **2nd degree:** Injury to the perineal muscle not involving the anal sphincter.
- **3rd degree:** Injury to the perineum and anal sphincter complex.
  - **3a:** Less than 50% of external anal sphincter (EAS).
  - **3b:** More than 50% of EAS.
  - **3c:** Internal anal sphincter (IAS) torn.
- **4th degree:** Injury to perineum involving the anal sphincter complex (EAS and IAS) and the rectal mucosa.

3rd and 4th degree perineal tears can be very debilitating as it can result in sexual dysfunction and faecal incontinence. 1st and 2nd degree tears can usually be repaired after delivery by trained midwives. 3rd and 4th degree tears are likely to require repair in theatre by an obstetrician.

5. E

Surgical management of pelvic organ prolapse is offered if non-surgical treatment is ineffective or unacceptable. The type of prolapse affects which procedure is most appropriate. This patient has a cystourethrocele in which there is a prolapse of the anterior vaginal wall, involving the bladder and urethra. The most appropriate option for this type of prolapse is an anterior repair, in which the bladder is pushed back into its normal anatomical position and the supporting tissue between the anterior wall of the vagina and the bladder is reinforced with sutures. A posterior repair is a similar procedure that is used to reinforce the connective tissue between the posterior wall of the vagina and the rectum and is, therefore, used to treat rectoceles.

The other three surgical procedures are used to treat either vaginal vault or uterine prolapse. Vaginal sacrospinous fixation involves suturing the top of the vagina to the sacrospinous ligament and is used to treat both vaginal vault and uterine prolapse. Similarly, vaginal sacrospinous hysteropexy involves suturing the cervix to the sacrospinous ligament and is used to treat uterine prolapse. An alternative procedure to treat uterine prolapse is vaginal hysterectomy. Finally, sacrocolpopexy involves using a mesh to attach the vaginal vault to the sacrum and is used to treat vaginal vault prolapse.

6. C

HELLP syndrome is a complication that mainly occurs in patients with pre-eclampsia. HELLP is a biochemical diagnosis that is based on the changes that are responsible for its name: **H**aemolysis, **E**levated **L**FTs and **L**ow **P**latelets. Patients who develop HELLP may also present with other signs of severe pre-eclampsia such as visual disturbances, epigastric pain, or an intense headache. Although the pathophysiology of HELLP syndrome is not fully understood, it is thought to result from endothelial injury which leads to fibrin deposition and haemolysis. It is important to identify HELLP syndrome early as it is associated with an increased risk of several complications including placental abruption and maternal death. The only definitive management option is expedited delivery of the baby. It is important to note that ALP is always high in pregnancy as it is produced by the placenta. Furthermore, a mild reduction in haemoglobin and a rise in MCV are also normal in pregnancy.

Obstetric cholestasis usually presents with itching of the hands and feet which is worst at night. Acute fatty liver of pregnancy presents with vague symptoms such as nausea, vomiting and abdominal pain, but patients may also develop jaundice and a fever. Biliary colic is caused by obstruction of the bile duct by a gallstone and presents with right upper quadrant pain that may be exacerbated by eating fatty meals. Cholecystitis will also present with right upper quadrant pain, and patients may also have a fever and jaundice. Reduced emptying of the gallbladder means that biliary conditions are more common in pregnancy.

7. B

The copper intrauterine device (IUD) is a form of long-acting reversible contraception that can also be used as emergency contraception if inserted within 120 hours of unprotected sexual intercourse. The copper coil is non-hormonal and, hence, does not cause oestrogenic or progestogenic side-effects. It can provide long-term contraception for up to 10 years. However, patients receiving the IUD need to be warned that periods may be heavier, longer, and more painful for the first 3–6 months. All intrauterine devices also carry a risk of uterine perforation and infection. Furthermore, patients have an increased risk of ectopic pregnancy.

The levonorgestrel intrauterine system (LNG-IUS) is another effective form of long-acting reversible contraception. It is often used to treat menorrhagia and dysmenorrhoea as it tends to make periods lighter, shorter, and less painful. However, as the IUS releases progesterone, some women experience hormonal side-effects such as acne, breast tenderness, decreased libido, mood changes, headaches, and nausea. These side-effects may also occur with the progesterone-only pill, contraceptive implant, and contraceptive injection. Women receiving a progesterone-based contraceptive should be warned that periods may become irregular or stop altogether. The contraceptive injection may cause a delay in the return of fertility of up to one year.

8. D

Epilepsy is a condition in which patients have a tendency to experience recurrent unprovoked seizures. It is an important comorbidity to monitor closely in pregnancy as it is associated with an increase in maternal mortality. Before a patient becomes pregnant, it is important to aim to reduce medication to monotherapy, where possible, and titrate the medication based on seizure frequency. Patients should be made aware of the teratogenic effects of antiepileptic drugs (e.g. neural tube defects, facial clefts, and cardiac defects) but they should also be made aware of the risks of uncontrolled epilepsy in pregnancy (maternal and foetal hypoxia). As this patient has had several seizures in the past 12 months, it would be prudent to continue antiepileptic medication. Furthermore, many antiepileptic drugs will cause a folic acid deficiency so patients with epilepsy should receive 5 mg folic acid as opposed to the standard 400 µg folic acid. Folic acid deficiency can result in neural tube defects such as spina bifida and anencephaly.

9. C

Causes of pruritus vulvae (itchy vulva) can be divided into non-neoplastic and neoplastic. Non-neoplastic conditions include lichen vulval dermatoses (e.g. lichen sclerosus, vulval dermatitis, lichen planus, and vulval psoriasis), infection (e.g. candidiasis, trichomoniasis, threadworms), and menopause (atrophic vaginitis). Neoplastic conditions include squamous vulval intraepithelial neoplasia (VIN) and vulval carcinoma. Lichen sclerosus is a chronic condition with unknown aetiology that most commonly occurs in post-menopausal women and tends to affect the genital and perianal areas. It presents with crinkled or thickened patches of skin that may be localised or may be more extensive, involving the clitoral hood, labia minora, and perianal skin in a figure of eight pattern. Importantly, lichen sclerosus never involves the vaginal mucosa. The lesions can be very itchy and sore, causing dysuria and dyspareunia, and leading to complications, such as phimosis of the clitoris and introital stenosis. Topical steroids are the mainstay of treatment.

Lichen sclerosus increases the risk of developing vulval intraepithelial neoplasia (VIN) and vulval squamous cell carcinoma. VIN refers to a precancerous skin lesion (squamous cell carcinoma *in situ*) that may cause vulval itching and burning with well-defined, flat and erythematous lesions. Most cases are associated with HPV infection. VIN is not invasive but may evolve into vulval cancer (squamous cell carcinoma). Vulval cancer also presents with itching or pain, but there may be an obvious wart-like nodule or ulcer present. VIN and vulval cancer tend to affect post-menopausal women. Vulvovaginal candidiasis presents with vulval itching with a thick, white vaginal discharge. Atrophic vulvovaginitis is thinning of the genital tissues due to oestrogen deficiency following menopause. It presents with dryness, itching, dyspareunia, vaginal spitting and thin, pale vulva that may split.

10. E

A low-lying placenta is defined as a placenta which is within 2 cm of the internal cervical os when viewed on a transabdominal ultrasound. It is important to identify a low-lying placenta at this stage as it allows monitoring later in pregnancy to identify placenta praevia. Women identified as having a low-lying placenta at 20 weeks should have another transabdominal ultrasound scan at 32 weeks. If the placenta is still low, a further scan should be arranged at 36 weeks. If, at 36 weeks, the placenta is low, an elective caesarean section is necessary as the cervical os is obstructed by the placenta. As the uterus grows upwards and outwards throughout pregnancy, it is likely that most low-lying placentas will move upwards and away from the internal cervical os with advancing gestation. Only around 10% of women with low-lying placentas will end up with placenta praevia, which requires an elective caesarean section. Nonetheless, it is important to rescan at these intervals and to take precautions (e.g. avoiding sex) if the placenta remains low, as it could precipitate a massive haemorrhage.

CTGs are unreliable at such an early gestation. Furthermore, bleeding in placenta praevia tends to be mostly maternal, and the foetal trace may not show any abnormalities in the presence of a bleeding placenta praevia. Antenatal corticosteroids will be futile at this gestation as the pregnancy is still below the threshold for viability.

11. C

Myomectomy is the only surgical procedure for fibroids that is fertility preserving. It is either done via laparotomy, laparoscopy or hysteroscopy depending on the size, location, and number of fibroids. Goserelin acetate is a gonadotrophin-releasing hormone (GnRH) analogue that causes ovarian suppression. Since fibroids are oestrogen-dependent, GnRH analogues lead to shrinking of fibroids and may be used before a myomectomy or hysterectomy. Patients need to be warned that goserelin acetate causes a temporary menopausal state and, therefore, use is limited to 3 months to prevent a dramatic reduction in bone mineral density. An alternative agent is ulipristal acetate (a progesterone antagonist) which can be also be used before surgery or intermittently in women who are not eligible for surgery. It needs to be given with caution as it can cause liver damage so regular monitoring of LFTs is required.

Hysterectomy is the most definitive way of treating fibroids. However, since fertility needs to be preserved, it would not be appropriate in this case. Hysteroscopic resection of fibroids is a surgical method used to remove submucosal fibroids. Endometrial ablation is a procedure that involves destroying the lining of the uterus with a heated wire. Although effective in treating heavy menstrual bleeding, pregnancy is not recommended after the procedure due to the increased risk of miscarriage and ectopic pregnancy. Uterine artery embolization is a radiological procedure that is useful in women with fibroids who are not eligible for surgery or would like to preserve their fertility.

12. A

Patients considered at high risk of pre-eclampsia should receive preventative treatment with 150 mg aspirin from 12 weeks' gestation until delivery. Patients with any one of the following major risk factors should receive treatment:

- Chronic kidney disease
- Hypertensive disease during a previous pregnancy
- Autoimmune diseases (e.g. systemic lupus erythematosus)
- Diabetes mellitus
- Chronic hypertension

Patients with two or more moderate risk factors (listed in the following) should also receive preventative treatment:

- Primiparity
- Advanced maternal age (>40 years)
- Pregnancy interval of more than 10 years
- BMI >35 kg/m^2 at booking visit
- Family history of pre-eclampsia
- Multiple pregnancy

All women should be screened for pre-eclampsia at every antenatal visit by measuring blood pressure and performing a urine dipstick. Please note that previous guidelines recommended 75 mg aspirin for the prevention of pre-eclampsia.

13. C

Premature ovarian insufficiency (POI) is a term used to describe menopause occurring before the age of 40 years. It is a biochemical diagnosis based on the results of a hormone profile. Ovarian failure results in a low oestradiol level and a consequent increase in FSH and LH due to the loss of negative feedback on the hypothalamus and pituitary gland. POI is diagnosed after a patient is found to have two FSH measurement above 30 U/L taken 4–6 weeks apart. POI is usually idiopathic, but primary causes include chromosomal abnormalities (e.g. Turner's syndrome) and autoimmune diseases. Secondary causes include infections (e.g. tuberculosis, malaria and mumps), chemotherapy, radiotherapy, and surgical menopause (e.g. bilateral oophorectomy). The main symptom of POI is amenorrhoea, but some women experience menopausal symptoms, such as hot flushes, night sweats, vaginal dryness, and mood swings. Midluteal progesterone is a measure of ovulation and will be low in patients with POI as they are not ovulating.

Polycystic ovarian syndrome (PCOS) will show an elevated LH and FSH with an LH:FSH ratio greater than 1:1. Furthermore, PCOS is also associated with hyperinsulinaemia which results in an elevated testosterone and reduced sex hormone binding globulin level. Hypogonadotrophic hypogonadism results from pituitary or hypothalamic insufficiency which can be congenital (e.g. Kallman syndrome) or acquired (e.g. eating disorders, excessive exercise, tumours). The blood results will show low FSH, LH, and oestradiol levels. Hyperprolactinaemia may be caused by functional prolactinomas, hypothyroidism (as TRH stimulates prolactin secretion) or dopamine antagonists such as antipsychotics (as dopamine inhibits prolactin secretion). Prolactin acts on the hypothalamus and reduces GnRH secretion, resulting in low FSH, LH, and oestradiol levels.

14. B

Symphysis-fundal height (SFH) is measured at every antenatal appointment from 24 weeks onwards. The SFH in centimetres should be equal to the gestational age in weeks (±2 cm). A lower than expected SFH should be followed up by an ultrasound scan to measure estimated foetal weight (EFW). EFW is based on four main parameters: abdominal circumference, head circumference, femur length, and biparietal diameter. Intrauterine growth restriction (IUGR) is defined as the failure of a foetus to maintain its expected growth rate. It can be classified as symmetrical and asymmetrical. Symmetrical growth restriction is typically caused by intrauterine infections and congenital syndromes which result in failure of appropriate growth of both the head and the abdomen (i.e. head and abdominal circumference will both be lower than expected). Asymmetrical growth restriction is usually caused by placental insufficiency and occurs later in pregnancy, resulting in sparing of head circumference with failure of growth of the abdomen as the foetus diverts its resources to preserve the brain. Asymmetrical growth restriction requires close monitoring as continued placental insufficiency could result in intrauterine death. Serial growth scans should be performed every 2 weeks and Doppler ultrasound scans should be performed twice-weekly.

15. D

Guidelines for the management of ectopic pregnancy can be seen on **Obstetrics and Gynaecology: Paper 2 Answers Section, No. 15**. Since this patient is symptomatic and has an adnexal mass greater than 35 mm in diameter with a visible foetal heartbeat, she requires surgical management. Laparoscopy is generally preferred to laparotomy as it is associated with reduced blood loss and faster recovery. Salpingectomy (removal of the fallopian tube) is preferred to salpingotomy (removing the affecting portion of the fallopian tube with anastomosis of the loose ends) to prevent recurrence. However, in the presence of contralateral tubal disease, as seen in this case, salpingotomy is preferred to preserve fertility. As this patient is haemodynamically stable, an urgent laparotomy is unnecessary.

16. A

A number of physiological changes take place in pregnancy to provide the ideal conditions for growth and development of the foetus and reduce the risk of complications (e.g. bleeding) at birth. The main changes are summarised based on organ system in the following table.

System	Changes in pregnancy
Haematology	Decreased Hb Increased MCV Increased plasma volume Increased neutrophils Decreased platelets Increased fibrinogen, factor VIII and vWF Decreased protein S
Respiratory	Increased tidal volume Same respiratory rate Increased oxygen consumption
Cardiovascular	Increased heart rate Increased stroke volume
Renal	Increased glomerular filtration rate
Gastrointestinal	Decreased intestinal tone and motility Decreased lower oesophageal sphincter tone Decreased gallbladder contractions

17. E

Women will require contraception after day 21 postpartum. The LNG-IUS is an effective and safe form of contraception but it can only be inserted within 48 hours of delivery or after 4 weeks. It is effective immediately after insertion.

Lactational amenorrhoea is 98% effective as a form of contraception provided that the woman is exclusively breastfeeding, amenorrhoeic, and within 6 months postpartum. Progestogens (e.g. implant, injection, pill) can be started at any point postpartum. If it is started after day 21, additional contraception should be used for the first 2 days. A small amount of progestogens enters the breastmilk, however, this is not harmful to the baby. The combined oral contraceptive pill (COCP) is contraindicated in women who are breastfeeding and less than 6 weeks postpartum as it can affect milk production. In women who are not breastfeeding, the COCP can be started from day 21.

18. D

Uterine hyperstimulation is defined as a uterine contraction frequency of more than 5 in 10 minutes or a single contraction lasting longer than 2 minutes. It is a complication of induced labour, hence why continuous CTG monitoring is necessary for all cases of induction of labour. It is important to identify and treat uterine hyperstimulation promptly as it can lead to foetal hypoxia and concerning foetal heart rate changes that require an emergency caesarean section. Uterine hyperstimulation caused by prostaglandins should be treated by administering a tocolytic such as terbutaline (b_2-agonist). If it is caused by excessive use of syntocinon, it may be managed by reducing or stopping the infusion.

Please refer to **Obstetrics and Gynaecology: Paper 1, Answers Section, No. 27; Obstetrics and Gynaecology: Paper 2, Answers Section, No. 18** for more information on the induction of labour and the conditions necessary for an instrumental delivery.

19. B

A characteristic feature of polycystic ovarian syndrome (PCOS) is anovulation. This leads to persistently elevated levels of oestrogen which promotes endometrial proliferation and can lead to the development of endometrial hyperplasia and cancer. Furthermore, a reduced frequency of endometrial shedding contributes to this increased risk. To reduce the risk of developing endometrial hyperplasia and cancer, patients with PCOS who are taking the combined oral contraceptive pill are recommended to have a withdrawal bleed at least every 3–4 months. Although some studies have suggested a potential increased risk of breast and ovarian cancer, this is somewhat contentious and PCOS is much more strongly associated with endometrial cancer. Other complications of PCOS include type 2 diabetes mellitus, cardiovascular disease, obesity, and obstructive sleep apnoea.

20. A

Pelvic girdle pain (previously known as symphysis pubis dysfunction) is a common musculoskeletal condition that occurs in pregnancy due to excessive movement of the pubic symphysis as the cartilage becomes lax under the influence of various pregnancy hormones (e.g. relaxin). It typically presents with pain and tenderness over the pubic symphysis which may spread to the back, thighs, and perineum. The pain is often worse when walking or climbing the stairs, and patients may mention that they can hear a clicking or grinding sound coming from their pelvis. Despite being painful to the mother, symphysis pubis dysfunction is not harmful to the baby, and can be treated with analgesia and physiotherapy.

Sciatica is a condition in which patients experience shooting pains along the distribution of the sciatic nerve. It is usually caused by spinal disc prolapse pressing on nerve roots. It is also relatively common in pregnancy. Braxton Hicks contractions are mild uterine contractions that typically occur from the second trimester onwards to prepare the uterine smooth muscle for labour. Sacroiliitis is inflammation of the sacroiliac joint and is usually associated with ankylosing spondylitis. Patients may complain of pain that wakes them up at night and pain when seated for a prolonged period. Spinal disc prolapse causes back pain with shooting pains along the legs. The straight leg raise is a useful clinical tool for identifying disc prolapse.

21. B

Pelvic inflammatory disease (PID) is an infection that typically arises in the vagina and spreads to the upper reproductive tract, involving the uterus, fallopian tubes, and ovaries. It is most commonly caused by *Chlamydia trachomatis* and *Neisseria gonorrhoea*. Other implicated organisms include *Mycoplasma genitalium* and commensal vaginal flora. Patients may present with lower abdominal pain, vaginal discharge, dyspareunia, and abnormal vaginal bleeding (intermenstrual or post-coital). A speculum examination may reveal cervicitis and a bimanual examination may elicit cervical excitation. Endocervical and high vaginal swabs may reveal the offending organisms. An FBC and CRP are useful for demonstrating raised inflammatory markers. If the patient is febrile, blood cultures should also be taken. PID can damage structures within the reproductive tract, in particular, the fallopian tubes, thereby increasing the risk of ectopic pregnancies in the future. It can also increase the risk of subfertility and chronic pelvic pain. PID should be promptly treated with antibiotics in accordance with trust guidelines to cover gonorrhoea, chlamydia, and Gram-negative organisms (e.g. IM ceftriaxone, oral doxycycline, and oral metronidazole). Pregnant women with PID and particularly severe cases should be treated with IV antibiotics. STI screening and contact tracing should also be offered to all patients.

22. A

Amniocentesis is a potential sensitising event in rhesus-negative women, so it requires prophylactic treatment with anti-D immunoglobulin. Anti-D immunoglobulin works by coating foetal red cells that have leaked into the maternal circulation, leading to their destruction by the lymphoreticular system. This prevents the maternal immune system from being sensitised to the rhesus D antigen present on the foetal red cells. Rhesus-negative women are routinely offered prophylactic anti-D either as a single dose (1500 IU) at 28 weeks, or two doses (500 IU) at 28 and 34 weeks. Prophylactic anti-D should also be given within 72 hours of any potential sensitising event. Potential sensitising events before 20 weeks include CVS, amniocentesis, abdominal trauma, and miscarriage. This is treated by giving a minimum of 250 IU anti-D immunoglobulin. Before 12 weeks, it is generally thought that the foetal blood volume is so low that sensitising events are unlikely, however, 250 IU anti-D immunoglobulin should be given for any surgical termination of pregnancy, surgical management of miscarriage or ectopic pregnancy and any molar pregnancy.

After 20 weeks, a 500 IU dose is used. A Kleihauer test should also be performed for any sensitising event after 20 weeks. It measures the volume of foetal blood that has entered the maternal circulation, thereby determining whether more anti-D immunoglobulin needs to be given.

23. E

All women with PMS should be offered lifestyle advice that include dietary modification (i.e. regular, balanced meals), regular exercise, sleep hygiene, stress reduction, and alcohol and smoking advice. For women with moderate severity symptoms, a continuous oral contraceptive pill may be used with cognitive behavioural therapy (CBT) if there are prominent mood symptoms. Women with severe symptoms may be given a selective serotonin reuptake inhibitor (SSRI) which can be taken continuously or just during the luteal phase. SSRIs tend to be most effective when taken in combination with CBT. Severity of PMS is determined by degree of impairment on professional and social function — this patient's PMS can be described as severe as she is missing work and social events due to her symptoms.

Patients should be advised that there is limited evidence to support the use of complementary treatments such as acupuncture, calcium and vitamin D supplements, ginkgo biloba, and evening primrose oil.

24. D

Preterm prelabour rupture of membranes (PPROM) is defined as the rupture of membranes before 37 weeks' gestation without the concurrent onset of labour. Patients typically complain of a sudden gush of fluid from the vagina. It is investigated by performing a sterile speculum examination which will reveal pooling of fluid. If this test is negative, testing for the presence of insulin-like growth factor (IGF) binding protein-1 and alpha-microglobulin-1 in the vaginal fluid may be considered. These tests have a high negative predictive value so are useful for ruling out PPROM.

The main issue with PPROM is the risk of developing an infection which can lead to significant morbidity or foetal death. To reduce the risk of infection, oral erythromycin should be commenced. Decisions about when to deliver is based on balancing the risks of preterm delivery with the risk of developing an intrauterine infection. This patient should be admitted for monitoring, started on antibiotics and IM corticosteroids may also be administered if delivery is likely to occur soon. Patients may be offered 24 hours of expectant management with antibiotic cover, as many women will spontaneously go into labour soon after rupturing their membranes. IV magnesium sulphate should be given if preterm delivery is expected within 24 hours or if preterm labour is established, as it has a neuroprotective effect on the baby. Foetal monitoring with a cardiotocograph (CTG) and advising the mother to pay close attention to foetal movements is essential, as it will be the basis of many decisions regarding the delivery.

25. C

Gestational trophoblastic disease is a spectrum of disease characterised by abnormal proliferation of pregnancy-associated trophoblast tissue. Diseases that fall under this umbrella term include complete and partial moles, invasive moles, and choriocarcinoma. The difference between complete and partial moles is based on the pathogenesis. Complete moles are formed when an egg containing no genetic material gets fertilised by either two sperm cells or one sperm cell followed by duplication of the genetic material of the sperm cell. Partial moles form when a normal egg is fertilised by two sperm cells or one sperm cell with unreduced paternal chromosomal material (46XY). The excess male chromosomes drive proliferation. Molar pregnancies typically present with irregular vaginal bleeding in early pregnancy, hyperemesis, a large-for-dates uterus, and hypertension. Key investigations include an ultrasound scan (which will reveal a 'snowstorm' or 'cluster of grapes' appearance) and serum β-hCG (likely to be elevated out of proportion with gestation). Patients may also develop symptoms of hyperthyroidism as β-hCG, at high concentrations, can act on TSH receptors.

Around 10% of complete moles will develop into locally invasive moles that can cause considerable damage to surrounding structures and 2.5% of complete moles will transform into a choriocarcinoma, which is a rapidly invasive, widely metastasising malignancy. Suspected molar pregnancies should be treated promptly with suction curettage — a surgical procedure that involves using suction to evacuate the contents of the uterus. This should be followed by serial β-hCG measurements to ensure that the mole does not persist. Although the clinical features and ultrasound findings can suggest a diagnosis of molar pregnancy, it can only be confirmed by histological analysis.

26. E

In a normal pregnancy, TSH levels will fall and free T4 levels will rise during the first trimester. To mimic this physiological rise in T4, patients who are being treated for hypothyroidism should increase their dose of levothyroxine by 25 μg per day even if they are currently euthyroid. Corrected hypothyroidism has no influence on pregnancy outcome or risk of complications. However, suboptimal replacement is associated with developmental delay and pregnancy loss. Women with hypothyroidism should continue thyroid replacement therapy throughout pregnancy and they should aim for biochemical euthyroidism (TSH <4 mU/L).

27. B

Cervical cancer is the second most common cancer in women worldwide. Mortality from cervical cancer is declining in the UK due to the cervical screening programme. Risk factors for cervical cancer include infection with human papilloma virus, the combined oral contraceptive pill, parity, smoking, and immunosuppression. There are two main types of cervical cancer: squamous cell carcinomas (70–80%) and adenocarcinomas (10%). The management of cervical cancer depends on its FIGO stage — summarised in the following table.

Stage	Description of tumour	Management
Stage 0	Carcinoma *in situ* (cervical intraepithelial neoplasia 3)	Large loop excision of the transformation zone (LLETZ)
Stage 1	Lesions confined to the cervix	
1A1	<3 mm deep and <7 mm across	Conservative management: cone biopsy, simple hysterectomy or simple trachelectomy

(Continued)

(*Continued*)

Stage	Description of tumour	Management
lA2	3–5 mm deep and <7 mm across	For tumours 4 cm or less, radical hysterectomy with lymphadenectomy is preferred to chemoradiation
lB1	Tumour <4 cm	
lB2	Tumour >4 cm	
Stage ll	Invasion beyond the uterus, but not into the pelvic wall or lower third of the vagina	For tumours larger than 4 cm, chemoradiation is preferred
llA	Invasion into upper 2/3 of vagina, but not parametrium	If fertility needs to be preserved, radical trachelectomy with lymphadenectomy may be considered instead
llA1	Tumour <4 cm	
llA2	Tumour >4 cm	
llB	Invasion into parametrium	Chemoradiation
Stage lll	Invasion into the pelvic wall and lower third of the vagina	
lllA	Involvement of the vagina but not the pelvic wall	
lllB	Involvement of the pelvic wall or non-functioning kidney	
Stage IV	Invasion of bladder or rectal mucosa	
lVA	Spread to adjacent pelvic organs	
lVB	Distant metastases	Combination chemotherapy or single agent therapy and palliative care

Radical hysterectomy involves removing the uterus, cervix, fallopian tubes, upper part of the vagina, and surrounding parametrium whereas radical trachelectomy is a fertility-sparing procedure that involves removing the cervix, upper part of the vagina and surrounding parametrium only. This patient's cancer is stage lB1 and, since fertility is not a priority, radical hysterectomy with lymphadenectomy is the most appropriate treatment option.

28. D

Caesarean sections are associated with a number of immediate complications (e.g. bleeding, infection, prolonged hospital stay) and it can have implications on future pregnancies. The caesarean section scar is considered a weak point in the wall of the uterus, thereby increasing the risk of uterine rupture during labour. This risk increases if patients have more caesarean sections. After one lower segment caesarean section, a vaginal birth after caesarean section (VBAC) has fewer complications than an elective repeat of caesarean section (ERCS). The risk of uterine rupture in patients having a VBAC after one previous lower segment caesarean section is low, however, the risk increases with the use of syntocinon. Patients will also have an increased risk of needing instrumental delivery for failure to progress. Features of a pregnancy that are favourable for VBAC include singleton pregnancies, cephalic presentation, more than 37 weeks' gestation, and only one previous lower segment caesarean section. With two or more previous caesarean sections, an ERCS is generally recommended but VBAC may be possible after discussion with a senior obstetrician. Contraindications for VBAC include previous uterine rupture, classical caesarean section scar (longitudinal midline incision as opposed to transverse), and contraindications that are unrelated to previous caesarean sections (e.g. placenta praevia).

29. B

Sudden onset lower abdominal pain with transvaginal ultrasound scan findings of free fluid around the ovary in a patient with a negative pregnancy test is suggestive of an ovarian cyst accident. Ovarian cysts are common in women of reproductive age and are often asymptomatic. They can, however, cause bloating and discomfort during sex. A cyst may rupture leading to severe acute lower abdominal pain. It is important to perform a pregnancy test as soon as possible as it can be difficult to clinically distinguish from an ectopic pregnancy. In the case of cyst rupture, the patient should be admitted for observation and given adequate analgesia. The pain should settle over 4–6 hours and a repeat transvaginal ultrasound scan should be arranged if there is any concern about ongoing bleeding.

Ovarian torsion is another complication of ovarian cysts which occurs when the ovary twists on a vascular pedicle, leading to ischaemia and, if untreated, necrosis of the ovary. A transvaginal ultrasound scan would reveal an oedematous ovary surrounded by free-fluid, sometimes referred to as 'whirlpool' sign. Ovarian torsion would require an emergency laparoscopy to detort the affected ovary. IV antibiotics are unnecessary as this is not an infectious process. Serum β-hCG would not be necessary as the pregnancy test is negative.

30. C

Gravidity and parity are frequently used terms in obstetrics and determining a patient's gravidity and parity can be surprisingly difficult in some circumstances. Gravidity refers to the number of times a woman has been pregnant, irrespective of the outcome of the pregnancy (i.e. a pregnancy carried to term, a termination of pregnancy and a miscarriage will each count as 1 in terms of gravidity). Parity refers to the number of foetuses delivered after a viable gestation (24 weeks). For example, a baby born prematurely at 28 weeks and a stillbirth at 28 weeks will each count as 1 in terms of parity. Multiple pregnancies make matters slightly more complicated. A twin pregnancy will count as 1 in terms of gravidity (as, although there are two foetuses, it is a single pregnancy) but, if delivered after a viable gestation, it will count as 2 in terms of parity. This patient has been pregnant 5 times in total (miscarriage + termination + stillbirth + twin pregnancy + current pregnancy) and she has delivered 3 foetuses beyond a viable gestation (twins + stillbirth) — therefore, she is G5 P3.

Psychiatry: Paper 1

Questions

1. A 25-year-old man has come to see his GP after having some trouble at work. He has recently started working at a bank and has found himself feeling increasingly anxious. He is particularly nervous about a presentation he needs to give in 2 weeks' time to some of his colleagues. On further questioning, he is worried about blushing and embarrassing himself in front of his new colleagues and has excused himself from several work socials. What is the most likely diagnosis?

   A Generalised anxiety disorder
   B Social phobia
   C Acute stress reaction
   D Agoraphobia
   E Panic disorder

2. A 7-year-old boy is brought to see the GP by his mother after his school expressed some concern about his performance. For the past 2 months, he has had issues concentrating in class and is easily distracted. He has also had difficulty sitting still and taking turns. His mother said that he has had no such issues at home. What is the most appropriate management option?

    A Watchful waiting
    B Parent training programme
    C Cognitive behavioural therapy
    D Methylphenidate
    E Fluoxetine

3. A 54-year-old patient with severe treatment-resistant depression has been referred for electroconvulsive therapy (ECT). He is concerned about the long-term consequences of the treatment. Which of the following is a long-term side-effect of ECT?

    A Impaired memory
    B Cardiac arrhythmia
    C Tension headache
    D Musculoskeletal pain
    E Lower seizure threshold

4. An 82-year-old care home resident has been admitted to hospital after he assaulted a carer. He had become increasingly agitated over the last few days and was exclaiming that he needed to escape the desert island. In hospital, he is oriented in time, space, and person but has no recollection of the event. He has had no other symptoms and has no past medical history. What is the most appropriate initial investigation to perform?

    A CT head scan
    B Pulse oximetry
    C Urine dipstick
    D Chest X-ray
    E Blood glucose level

5. A 75-year-old woman, with a history of schizoaffective disorder, is prescribed a course of haloperidol. Her delusions reduce in frequency and intensity. Three weeks after beginning treatment, a mental health nurse noticed that she is stamping her feet and wringing her wrists

during a home visit. She mentions that she has been feeling restless. What is the most appropriate next step in her management?

A Start on zopiclone
B Start on propranolol
C Start on procyclidine
D Reduce dose of haloperidol
E Switch to clozapine

6. A 24-year-old woman comes to see her GP asking for a sick note for work. She has taken 3 days off work as she feels anxious about underperforming in her job as a salesperson. She feels that all the other salespeople are much better than her and she fears she will lose her job if her boss discovers that she is underperforming. She was previously made redundant by her last employer after having too much time off. What is the most likely diagnosis?

A Generalised anxiety disorder
B Social phobia
C Avoidant personality disorder
D Paranoid personality disorder
E Dependent personality disorder

7. A 31-year-old man presents to his GP with aching muscles and joints. He has also felt feverish and has had three bouts of diarrhoea this morning. On examination, he is sweaty and has dilated pupils. He denies any drug use or previous psychiatric history and says he just wants some 'strong painkillers' to make him feel better. What is the most likely diagnosis?

A Delirium tremens
B Cocaine intoxication
C Cocaine withdrawal
D Benzodiazepine withdrawal
E Opioid withdrawal

8. A 33-year-old man has been suffering with a low mood for the past 6 months. He cannot identify any particular trigger and recalls suffering from similar prolonged episodes in the past. He complains of feeling tired all the time and has become increasingly socially isolated and is struggling at work. He is particularly bothered by his difficulty getting to sleep and his loss of appetite. He would like to receive treatment to ameliorate these issues whilst he is on the waiting list for CBT. What is the most appropriate treatment option?

    A Mirtazapine
    B Sertraline
    C Citalopram
    D Fluoxetine
    E Venlafaxine

9. A 29-year-old cannabis user has become deeply anxious and distressed over the last 6 months. He often locks himself in his apartment and refuses to leave for weeks at a time. He mentions that he regularly hears a muffled, distant voice of an alien from Mars saying, 'I'm coming for you'. What is this psychiatric phenomenon?

    A Pareidolic illusion
    B Thought echo
    C Command hallucination
    D Extracampine hallucination
    E Elemental hallucination

10. A 45-year-old man attends an outpatient psychiatry appointment complaining of having several distressing episodes in which he visualises images of child pornography. He recognises the images as coming from within his own mind and has started self-harming whenever he sees these images to try and prevent them from happening. He has never had any sexual thoughts about children before and has avoided social situations since this problem started as he feels embarrassed about his 'perversion'. What is the most likely diagnosis?

A Disorder of sexual preference
B Schizophrenia
C Schizoid personality disorder
D Obsessive compulsive disorder
E Delusional disorder

11. A 76-year-old woman is receiving treatment for a UTI on the care of the elderly ward. She has made several comments about wanting to end her life. Her husband passed away 3 weeks ago, and she said that she is going to jump on the railway tracks near the hospital. She has removed her drip and is threatening to leave the ward. On assessment, she has capacity but seems severely depressed. A decision is made to section her under the Mental Health Act. Which section would be the most appropriate in this scenario?

A Section 2
B Section 3
C Section 5(2)
D Section 5(4)
E Section 135

12. A 14-year-old girl is referred to CAMHS with concerns about her body weight. She complains of feeling fat and is terrified of gaining weight. She admits to skipping meals and regularly using laxatives. On examination, she is emaciated, dehydrated, and has lanugo hair. She is bradycardic and has a postural drop. Given the most likely diagnosis, what is the most appropriate management for this patient?

A CBT
B MANTRA
C SSCM
D Family therapy
E Start on sertraline

13. A 27-year-old man presents to A&E claiming he woke up with some abdominal pain and bloating and that he is researched his symptoms

and he is convinced that he has appendicitis. On examination, his abdomen is soft and non-tender and Rovsing's sign negative. His blood results and vital signs are all within the normal ranges. This is his ninth visit to A&E this year, and he has had several investigations which have never revealed a cause for concern. The patient becomes agitated when he is told that he is clinically well, and exclaims that he needs more investigations. What is the most likely diagnosis?

    A Conversion disorder
    B Dissociative disorder
    C Munchausen's syndrome
    D Somatisation disorder
    E Hypochondriasis

14. A patient currently undergoing CBT for depression has been prescribed a course of phenelzine. Which of the following foods should he be advised to avoid?

    A Shellfish
    B Eggs
    C Cheese
    D Peanuts
    E Milk

15. An 86-year-old man is seen in the outpatient clinic after his daughter expressed some concerns about his memory. He has become increasingly forgetful over the past 2 years. He often misplaces his belongings and forgets what he has done during the day. He recently left his gas hob on overnight which prompted his daughter to seek help. His long-term memory appears to be intact. He achieves a score of 22 on the Mini Mental State Examination. What is the most appropriate medication for this patient?

    A Rivastigmine
    B Memantine
    C Haloperidol

D Quetiapine

E Lorazepam

16. A 50-year-old woman presents to A&E with a fever and diarrhoea. On examination, her blood pressure is 166/122 mm Hg, her heart rate is 128 bpm, her reflexes are exaggerated, and her limbs appear to jerk on occasion. She has a past medical history of generalised anxiety disorder, which is being treated with sertraline. She admits that she tried cocaine at an office party last night. What is the most likely diagnosis?

    A Cocaine intoxication
    B Serotonin syndrome
    C Neuroleptic malignant syndrome
    D Discontinuation syndrome
    E Excited delirium

17. A 57-year-old man is brought into A&E by his brother. The patient says that he has been hearing a man's voice telling him that he is going to die. He claims he can see little people climbing up the wall and feels insects crawling over his arms and legs. On examination, he is emaciated, there is shifting dullness, yellowing of the sclera, and dilatation of the umbilical veins. He is sweaty, agitated, and a bilateral tremor is observed. His brother claims that he has a history of alcohol abuse, consuming up to 60 units per week. His vital signs are shown as follows:

Heart rate: 116 bpm
Blood pressure: 154/112 mm Hg
Respiratory rate: 24 breaths/min
Temperature: 37.1°C

What is the most likely underlying diagnosis?

    A Wernicke's encephalopathy
    B Korsakoff's syndrome
    C Alcoholic hallucinosis

    D Delirium tremens
    E Acute alcohol withdrawal

18. A 23-year-old woman has been referred to the psychiatry team with suspected schizophrenia after she has become increasingly socially withdrawn over the past year and has developed paranoid delusions of a man in hooded overalls visiting her house at night to murder her. She is known to the psychiatry services as she has previously suffered from anorexia nervosa and is steadily regaining weight despite her expressing concerns about her 'rapid' weight gain. What is the most appropriate management option?

    A Quetiapine
    B Mirtazapine
    C Olanzapine
    D Clozapine
    E Lithium

19. A 24-year-old man is being treated in A&E after presenting with deep cuts across his back. He seems reluctant to explain where they came from, but on further questioning, he eventually reveals that he asked his partner to whip him with a belt during sexual intercourse. He reveals that he gets sexual gratification from being in pain. What term is used to describe this sexual preference?

    A Fetishism
    B Paraphilia
    C Sadism
    D Masochism
    E Bondage

20. A 22-year-old man presents to his GP with a 2-year history of anxiety. He has found himself frequently ruminating about relatively small issues (such as road closures affecting his route to work). His sleep has suffered and his performance at work has deteriorated as he finds it difficult to focus on the task at hand. He has a past medical

history of type 1 diabetes mellitus and asthma. He has been referred for CBT but would like some medication to relieve his anxiety whilst he waits to start CBT. What is the most appropriate option?

    A Propranolol
    B Diazepam
    C Sertraline
    D Pregabalin
    E Fluoxetine

21. A 33-year-old survivor of a tsunami has been referred to psychiatry as he has read about post-traumatic stress disorder (PTSD) online and is worried that he might be experiencing it. Which of the following is a main feature of PTSD?

    A Flashbacks
    B Blunted startle reflex
    C Emotional instability
    D Symptoms lasting 2 weeks
    E Excessive sleep

22. A 27-year-old woman, with a history of bipolar I disorder, wishes to become pregnant but would like more information about the effects of her medication on the pregnancy. She has been stable on lithium and has only had one manic episode in the last 3 years. Which complication is lithium use in pregnancy associated with?

    A Cleft palate
    B Persistent pulmonary hypertension
    C Spina bifida
    D Ebstein's anomaly
    E Interrupted aortic arch

23. A 45-year-old man who lives with his family has recently resigned from his job as a software engineer to spend more time rebuilding the fence in his garden. He noticed that the fence was weathered and

asymmetrical a few months ago and decided that he would rebuild it to improve the aesthetic of his house. What is this psychiatric phenomenon?

A Mania
B Obsession
C Overvalued idea
D Delusion
E Compulsion

24. An ambulance has been called for a homeless man who was found unconscious at a bus stop. On examination, his pupils are constricted and his respiratory rate is 6 breaths/min. What is the first step in this patient's management?

A Admit for inpatient monitoring
B Administer IM naloxone
C Administer IM naltrexone
D Administer oral chlordiazapoxide
E Administer IV flumazenil

25. A 26-year-old woman is brought to A&E by the police after they found her walking down a busy road shouting at traffic. Her boy-friend is contacted to obtain a collateral history. He says that she has been behaving strangely for the last week. She has been claiming that she is from another planet and has been seeing little grey creatures following her. Her speech is confused and disorganised. She has recently lost her sister in a road traffic accident. What is the most likely diagnosis?

A Schizophrenia
B Manic episode
C Depressive episode
D Acute and transient psychosis
E Grief reaction

26. A 19-year-old girl comes into A&E after cutting her wrists with a butter knife. She explains that a new boyfriend, whom she's been on two dates with, cancelled their next date. This made her feel lonely and enraged so she messaged him saying that she is going to end her life and it will be his fault. Emotionally unstable personality disorder is suspected, and dialectical behavioural therapy (DBT) is recommended. How should DBT be explained to the patient?

   A It will teach you how your thoughts, feelings, and behaviours influence each other and that negative thoughts and feelings can trap you in a vicious cycle

   B It involves making side-to-side eye movements by following the movement of the therapist's finger while recalling traumatic events

   C It involves exploring the relationship between the therapist and client and allows you to understand how the past influences current behaviour

   D It teaches you how to accept who you are and how to deal with difficult emotions by recognising them and challenging them

   E It teaches you how to think about thinking and examine your own thoughts and beliefs and assess whether they are useful or realistic

27. A 21-year-old woman is currently being investigated for an eating disorder. She reports weekly episodes of eating several large pizzas and tubs of ice cream in one sitting, often followed by a feeling of intractable guilt which she relieves by forcefully vomiting. Her weight has remained relatively stable and she has a BMI of 20 kg/m². Which of the following is a complication of this disease?

   A Heavy periods
   B Dental caries
   C Hirsutism
   D Hyperkalaemia
   E Oesophageal dysmotility

28. A patient has been prescribed clozapine for treatment-resistant schizophrenia. Which of the following is most important to monitor in a patient taking clozapine?

    A Fasting blood glucose
    B Lipid profile
    C Neutrophil count
    D Sodium
    E Prolactin

29. A 30-year-old man presents with a 3-month history of low mood, sleep disturbance, and reduced appetite. He has also been feeling more tired than usual and no longer enjoys socialising with his friends. He is diagnosed with depression and started on sertraline. Which of the following side-effects might he experience?

    A Dry cough
    B Muscle spasms
    C Reduced sweating
    D Increased salivation
    E Erectile dysfunction

30. A 42-year-old man, with a history of schizoaffective disorder, becomes aggressive on the ward round. He attempts to attack a member of the nursing staff and is screaming offensive slurs. He is given a rapid tranquilisation of intramuscular lorazepam and haloperidol. Four hours later he becomes ataxic, his speech is slurred and his respiratory rate drops to 6 breaths/min. Given the most likely diagnosis, what is the first-line management option?

    A Administer intravenous naloxone
    B Administer oral activated charcoal
    C Administer oral diazepam
    D Administer intravenous flumazenil
    E Administer intravenous acetylcysteine

Answers

1. B

Social phobia is a type of phobic anxiety disorder that is characterised by a fear of scrutiny by other people leading to avoidance of social situations. Patients often complain that their main concern is embarrassing themselves in front of others.

Agoraphobia is a similar condition which is characterised by a fear of leaving home. This manifests as anxiety when in crowds and public places. Panic disorder is characterised by recurrent attacks of severe anxiety which are not restricted to any particular situation and are, therefore, unpredictable. Patients may complain of sudden-onset palpitations, chest pain, and a choking sensation. Generalised anxiety disorder describes anxiety that is persistent and not restricted to any particular environment, sometimes referred to as 'free floating' anxiety. Symptoms must be present for 6 months to be diagnostic. It is worth noting that any anxiety disorder can manifest with features of autonomic arousal (e.g. palpitations, sweating, tremor) so the diagnoses are primarily differentiated based on the triggers and pattern of symptoms. An acute stress reaction is a transient state that develops in response to extreme physical and mental stress. It typically manifests with a state of daze and disorientation which resolves after a few hours or days.

2. A

This patient has only had symptoms of inattention and hyperactivity for 2 months and the behaviour is restricted to one environment (i.e. at school). Therefore, this does not fit a diagnosis of attention deficit hyperactivity disorder (ADHD) which requires the presence of symptoms for at least 6 months in at least two different environments. In this situation, watchful waiting would be the best initial management plan. If the symptoms eventually meet the criteria for ADHD, treatment should be considered.

3. A

Electroconvulsive therapy (ECT) is used to treat catatonia, prolonged or severe manic episodes and severe life-threatening depression. It involves inducing a generalised tonic–clonic seizure in the patient under general anaesthesia. It was explored as a treatment option for depression after it was found that epileptic patients with depression reported an improvement in their mood after having a seizure. The main long-term side-effect of ECT is impaired memory. Short-term side-effects include cardiac arrhythmias, headaches, nausea, and muscle aches.

4. C

Delirium is an acute confusional state resulting from an organic cause. It is more common in elderly patients and common causes include infection, constipation, dehydration, and hypoxia. It typically has a fluctuating course, so patients may appear relatively lucid at certain intervals. Urinary tract infections are a common cause of delirium that may be asymptomatic. As it is very easy to perform a urine dipstick to rule out infection, this would be the most appropriate initial investigation to perform.

Pneumonia is another common infectious cause of delirium, however, the patient is likely to have respiratory symptoms such as a cough or shortness of breath. In patients with a history of diabetes mellitus, it is important to check their blood glucose as hypoglycaemia can cause delirium. Pulse oximetry is useful to rule out carbon monoxide poisoning, which should be suspected if several patients, who have been exposed to the same environment, present with delirium. Intracranial bleeds and strokes can present with delirium so a CT head scan may be useful, however, it should not be performed before simple bedside tests such as a urine dipstick.

5. B

Haloperidol is a typical antipsychotic agent. Whilst these agents are cheap and effective, they can also cause distressing extrapyramidal side-effects (EPSE) at therapeutic doses. This patient is describing akathisia — a feeling of constant restlessness which often makes patients want to move or shake their arms and legs. Akathisia can be treated with low-dose propranolol or lorazepam. The four types of EPSEs, their onset, symptoms, and treatment are listed in the following table.

Type of EPSE	Onset	Symptoms	Treatment
Dystonia	Early, sometimes within hours	An involuntary, painful, sustained muscle spasm e.g. oculogyric spasm, torticollis	Anticholinergic, e.g. procyclidine
Akathisia	Hours to weeks	An unpleasant feeling of restlessness; patients often have to pace about or jiggle their legs	Decrease dose or change antipsychotic. Propranolol or benzodiazepine
Parkinsonism	Days to weeks	Triad: resting tremor, rigidity and bradykinesia	Decrease dose or change antipsychotic. Anticholinergic, e.g. procyclidine
Tardive dyskinesia	Months to years	Rhythmic involuntary movements of the mouth, face, limbs, and trunk. Patients may grimace, make chewing, and sucking movements or excessively blinking. Often irreversible	Stop drug or reduce dose and switch to an atypical or clozapine Avoid anticholinergics as these may worsen the problem Tetrabenazine is used for moderate/severe

Zopiclone is a non-benzodiazepine 'Z drug' used in the short-term management of insomnia. It can only be prescribed for a short period of 2–4 weeks due to the risk of dependency. It is avoided in elderly patients due to an increased risk of falls. This patient has not complained of sleep disturbance and, therefore, zopiclone would not be appropriate. Procyclidine is an anti-cholinergic used to treat dystonia and Parkinsonism. Whilst reducing the dose of haloperidol is a possible answer, an effective therapeutic dose has been established and a reduction in dose may lead to a relapse in symptoms. Therefore, it is more appropriate to prescribe propranolol to control the side-effects. Clozapine is an atypical antipsychotic used for treatment-resistant schizophrenia. This patient has benefitted from haloperidol so is not considered treatment-resistant.

6. C

A personality disorder is characterised by problems in the way in which people handle their feelings resulting in issues with interpersonal interactions. They are often defined by the **3 Ps** — **P**ervasive (occurs in all/most areas of life), **P**ersistent (evident in adolescence and continues through adulthood), and **P**athological (causes distress to self or others and impairs functioning). Personality disorders are divided into 'clusters' which are listed as follows.

Cluster	Disorder	Features
A	Paranoid	Excessive sensitivity to setbacks Suspiciousness Tendency to distort experience to interpret neutral actions as hostile Combative sense of personal rights Excessive self-importance and self-reference
	Schizoid	Withdrawal from social contacts Preference for solitary activities Limited capacity to express feelings
	Schizotypal	Eccentric behaviour Bizarre thoughts not amounting to delusions Cold affect Tendency to social withdrawal
B	Antisocial	Disregard for social obligations Disregard for the feelings of others Behaviour is not modifiable by punishment Tendency to blame others
	Emotionally unstable	Tendency to act impulsively Mood instability Outbursts of emotion Tendency to quarrelsome behaviour
	Histrionic	Shallow and labile affect Exaggerated expression of emotion Egocentricity Lack of consideration of others Continuously seeking attention

(Continued)

(Continued)

Cluster	Disorder	Features
	Narcissistic	Grandiose sense of self-importance Belief that one is special Need for excessive admiration Lack of empathy Arrogance
C	Anankastic	Perfectionism Checking and preoccupation with details Unwelcome thoughts or impulses that do not meet the severity of OCD
	Avoidant	Feelings of tension and apprehension Insecurity and inferiority Yearning to be liked Sensitivity to rejection or criticism
	Dependent	Pervasive reliance on other people to make life decisions Fear of abandonment Feelings of helplessness and incompetence Passive compliance with the wishes of others

This patient demonstrates many of the features of avoidant personality disorder which include avoidance of work or social activities, anticipating criticism and disapproval, and concerns about being ridiculed or rejected.

Generalised anxiety disorder (GAD) is characterised by the presence of free-floating anxiety that is not restricted to any particular environment or circumstance. Symptoms have to be present for 6 months to be defined as GAD. The predominant feature of social phobia is a fear of scrutiny by other people which leads to avoidance of social situations. This can manifest as panic attacks when placed in uncomfortable social situations.

7. E
This patient has developed opioid withdrawal, which usually presents with generalised muscle and joint pains, abdominal cramps, fever, and 'everything runs' (i.e. diarrhoea, vomiting, lacrimation, and rhinorrhoea). These patients often appear agitated with dilated pupils and goosebumps. He may be falsely denying drug use in the hope of being prescribed an opioid to treat his symptoms. Symptoms usually start within 12 hours

of last heroin use and within 30 hours of last methadone use. Whilst these symptoms are very uncomfortable for the patient, they are not life-threatening. This is in contrast to delirium tremens — a form of alcohol withdrawal that occurs within 48–96 hours after last exposure to alcohol and presents with delirium, seizures, tremor, agitation, visual, auditory, and tactile hallucinations (classically seeing little people or animals, or feeling insects crawling over the skin) and autonomic dysfunction. Symptoms often appear suddenly and progress quickly. Seizures may occur without other symptoms of delirium tremens and may occur earlier (within 12–48 hours).

Benzodiazepine withdrawal presents similarly to alcohol withdrawal with symptoms such as sweating, insomnia, headache, tremor, nausea, and psychological features (anxiety, depression, and panic attacks). This occurs within several hours of the last exposure to a short-acting benzodiazepine. To prevent benzodiazepine withdrawal, patients who are dependent on benzodiazepines are switched onto diazepam (as it has a long half-life) and the dose is slowly tapered down over months. Cocaine intoxication creates a feeling of euphoria, but the side-effects include tachycardia, nausea, hypertension, dilated pupils, and hallucinations. Cocaine withdrawal occurs in two phases. Firstly, patients experience a crash, which occurs several hours after last use and is characterised by depression, exhaustion, agitation, and irritability. This is followed by a continuous withdrawal state featuring increasing cravings, irritability, lack of energy, poor concentration, insomnia, and slowed activity. This phase lasts between 1 and 10 weeks and carries a particularly high risk of relapse.

8. A
This patient has presented with several symptoms of depression which have been ongoing for several months. The lack of a trigger and recollection of previous similar episodes suggests that the root cause of the depression is more likely to be biochemical rather than psychosocial. The duration of the symptoms and its impact on his social and professional functioning suggests that his can be classified as moderate-to-severe depression. This warrants treatment with high-intensity psychological intervention (e.g. CBT or interpersonal therapy) and antidepressants. SSRIs (e.g. sertraline,

fluoxetine, and citalopram) are usually used as first-line antidepressants. Although they have the same mechanism of action, the choice between them may be influenced by patient factors. For example, sertraline is considered safest in patients who have comorbid medical conditions (especially if they have a history of ischaemic heart disease) and fluoxetine is the SSRI of choice in children and adolescents. Mirtazapine is a noradrenergic and specific serotoninergic antidepressant (NaSSA) which has a sedating effect that helps improve sleep and stimulate appetite. Therefore, it would be the most appropriate option in this case. Venlafaxine is a serotonin–noradrenaline reuptake inhibitor (SNRI) which is usually used if SSRIs are ineffective or unacceptable.

9. D

A hallucination is the perception of a sensation (e.g. visual, auditory, or tactile) without an external stimulus. There are several subtypes of hallucination. An extracampine hallucination is a hallucination that exceeds the limits of a normal sensory field. For example, in this scenario, it is impossible to hear a voice being projected from Mars.

An elemental hallucination are simple hallucinations such as flashes of light or noises. A command hallucination is a type of auditory hallucination in which voices speak to the patient in the second person (e.g. 'you should run in front of the traffic'). Thought echo is another type of auditory hallucination and one of Schneider's first rank symptoms of schizophrenia. The thoughts of the patient appear to be spoken out aloud. An illusion is an altered perception in which a real external object is falsely interpreted. It is usually heavily influenced by the affective state of the patient. For example, a patient who is anxious about walking through the street after dark may see a shadow of a lamppost and think that it is a person. A pareidolic illusion is when meaningful images are perceived from a vague stimulus (e.g. seeing a face in a fire).

10. D

Obsessive compulsive disorder (OCD) is a common mental health disorder characterised by the presence of recurrent intrusive thoughts or compulsive acts. Although common examples of obsessions typically involve excessive cleaning or checking, any recurrent thought or compulsion can be considered OCD, including ideas and images. Obsessional thoughts differ from delusions and psychoses in that they are distressing to the patient, recognised as their own despite being involuntary, and attempts are made to resist these thoughts. Furthermore, this patient shows no evidence of having any bizarre beliefs which are avidly held despite the presence of contradictory evidence. Delusional disorder is characterised by the presence of delusions in the absence of other psychotic phenomena (e.g. hallucinations). This is not a disorder of sexual preference as the patient clearly described having no sexual feelings towards children and the patient has shown clear distress about the mental images he has been seeing.

11. C

Sectioning is the act of detaining someone in hospital under the Mental Health Act 1983 and should only be done if:

- A patient needs to be assessed and treated for a mental health condition urgently.
- A patient's health would be at serious risk if treatment was not given urgently.
- The patient's or someone else's safety is at serious risk.
- The patient needs to be assessed and treated in hospital.

The most commonly used sections are outlined in the following table.

Section	Who by?	What for?	How long?
2	An approved mental health professional (AMPH) and two doctors one of whom is section 12 approved	The patient needs to be detained for assessment and possibly treatment	28 days The patient is often re-assessed to determine if section 3 is necessary
3	AMPH and two doctors one of whom is section 12 approved	The patient needs to be detained for treatment	6 months

(Continued)

(Continued)

Section	Who by?	What for?	How long?
4	AMPH and one doctor who is section 12 approved	Emergency power when there is a delay for a 2nd doctor and the patient needs to be detained for assessment	72 hours
5(2)	One doctor (can be non-psychiatric)	Holding power to detain inpatients for assessment; can be used on inpatients on any ward but cannot be used in A&E	72 hours
5(4)	One mental health nurse	Holding power to detain inpatient for consideration by a doctor of whether to use their 5(2) holding power or to arrange a Mental Health Act assessment	6 hours
17A	One doctor and AMPH	Community treatment order which allows patients under section to be treated safely in the community	If the conditions of the 17A are broken the patient may be detained in hospital
135	AMPH applies to the magistrate for a court order. Police enter the property with AMPH and doctor	Patient is physically removed from their home and detained for assessment	72 hours
136	Police	The police can transport a patient to their nearest place of safety if they are displaying a mental health disorder that requires urgent assessment and treatment	72 hours

This patient is suicidal and poses a serious risk to herself. It would therefore be inappropriate to allow her to leave hospital. A section 5(2) is most appropriate here as it is an emergency and there is insufficient time to organise a section 2. Under section 5(2), she would have a Mental Health Act assessment within 72 hours and may be subsequently detained under a section 2.

12. D

This patient fulfils the diagnostic criteria for anorexia nervosa: restriction of energy intake relative to requirement resulting in endocrine derangement (e.g. delayed puberty), intense fear of gaining weight, and a distorted body image. Other physical signs of anorexia nervosa include brittle hair and nails, peripheral cyanosis, Russel's sign (calluses on the knuckles from self-induced vomiting), swollen salivary glands, abdominal tenderness, dental caries, muscle wasting, short stature, and signs of hypercholesterolaemia and hypercarotenaemia.

Children and adults with anorexia nervosa are offered psychological treatment, dietary advice, and physical monitoring. Adults are offered one of three talking therapies: eating disorder-focused CBT, Maudsley Anorexia Nervosa Treatment for Adults (MANTRA) or Specialist Supportive Clinical Management (SSCM). MANTRA involves talking to a therapist to discover the root cause of the eating disorder and encouraging a behavioural change to develop a non-anorexic identity. SSCM is similar to MANTRA but is considered to be more practical. Patients are taught about nutrition and how certain eating habits contribute to physical symptoms. Focal psychodynamic therapy (FPT) can also be offered if these three treatments are ineffective. FPT involves exploring past experiences that may have contributed to the development of an eating disorder.

In children, the first-line management option is family therapy. The child is seen together with family members and treatment aims to emphasise the role of the family in helping the child recover. This also involves education on nutrition and the harmful effects of malnutrition. If family therapy is ineffective, CBT can be considered. SSRIs are generally not recommended for the treatment of anorexia nervosa in children, however, fluoxetine may be prescribed if the patient has co-existing depression or anxiety.

13. E

Hypochondriasis is a condition in which the patient has a persistent belief that he or she has a serious underlying disease. Such patients may refuse to accept negative test results and may become defensive if a doctor attempts to reassure them. Patients will typically have a specific disease that they are worried about (in this case, appendicitis). Somatisation is a slightly different disorder in which patients experience physical symptoms (e.g. abdominal pain) which is a manifestation of an underlying mental health disorder (e.g. anxiety). The symptoms are typically multiple, recurrent, and often changing, and should, by definition, last for more than 2 years to be classified as somatisation disorder.

Conversion disorder presents with an acute and severe impairment of motor or sensory function (e.g. paralysis, blindness, seizures, and numbness). It results from a psychological trigger (e.g. stress) rather than a physical issue. These patients exhibit la belle indifference — a lack of concern for the symptoms caused by a conversion disorder. Dissociative disorders involve a detachment from reality in order to escape from trauma. Patients feel disconnected from themselves and the world around them. Symptoms are closely associated with traumatic events and tend to last weeks to months. Like conversion disorder, no organic cause can be identified. There are three main presentations of dissociative disorder: disorders of movement or sensation, amnesia, and identity disorder (multiple personality disorder). All of the mentioned disorders are not factitious (i.e. the patient is not consciously feigning the symptoms to receive medical attention) or malingering (i.e. the patient is not feigning the symptoms for rewards such as a sick note or drugs). Munchausen's syndrome is a factitious disorder in which patients feign physical or psychological symptoms in order to receive medical attention and play the sick role.

14. C

Phenelzine is a monoamine oxidase inhibitor (MAOI), which inhibits the metabolism of monoamines thereby, causing an increase in their synaptic concentrations. There are two subclasses of MAOI: reversible and non-reversible. Phenelzine is a non-reversible agent, which covalently binds to the enzyme and blocks its activity. Non-reversible agents are associated with the 'cheese reaction' — an acute hypertensive attack which is caused by the reaction between MAOI and tyramine-rich foods (e.g. cheese). Such agents are rarely used because of the potential dangers of the cheese reaction. Reversible agents (e.g. moclobemide) are not associated with the cheese reaction. MAOIs can only be prescribed by mental health specialists and a 2-week washout period (free from other antidepressants) is required before non-reversible agents can be given.

MAOIs are not the first-line agents for depression and should only be considered after 3–4 weeks of treatment with a therapeutic dose of a first-line agent (usually an SSRI). Initially, a different SSRI may be attempted and then subsequently venlafaxine, a tricyclic antidepressant or a MAOI may be trialled. For moderate and severe depression, pharmacological therapy should be in combination with psychological therapy.

15. A

Alzheimer's disease is the most common cause of dementia and it presents with progressive loss of anterograde memory with intact long-term memory. Managing Alzheimer's disease (and any other form of dementia) requires a holistic approach. As Alzheimer's disease is an irreversible and incurable disease, the focus should be on preserving independence and quality of life. Several conservative adaptations should be considered to orient the patient (e.g. visible clocks and calendars) and to keep them safe (e.g. changing gas to electricity, door mat buzzers). They may also require social support to assist them with activities of daily living such as personal care, cooking, and cleaning. Patients with Alzheimer's disease may be subject to diagnostic overshadowing due to their diagnosis, so it is important to treat sensory impairments (e.g. with hearing aids), review their medication and exclude underlying delirium. Psychological therapies for

Alzheimer's disease include group cognitive stimulation and group reminiscence therapy. The activities are designed to train their memory and revisit distant memories. The first-line pharmacological treatment for mild-to-moderate Alzheimer's disease is an acetylcholinesterase inhibitor such as donepezil, rivastigmine, or galantamine. Although they do not change the course of the illness, they may provide symptomatic relief.

Memantine is an NMDA antagonist that is used in severe Alzheimer's disease or if acetylcholinesterase inhibitors are contraindicated or not tolerated. Patients with Alzheimer's disease may develop behavioural problems which require sedatives or antipsychotics as a last resort such as lorazepam, haloperidol, and quetiapine.

16. B

Serotonin syndrome is a constellation of symptoms caused by high levels of serotonin usually due to misuse of drugs that cause an increase in serotonin concentration (e.g. SSRIs). It typically causes a fever, hypertension, tachycardia, agitation, diarrhoea, hyperreflexia, and myoclonus. It tends to happen when two or more drugs that raise serotonin levels are taken together (in this case, sertraline and cocaine). Other drugs that can cause serotonin syndrome include all classes of antidepressants, triptans, St John's wort, lithium, metoclopramide, and other illicit drugs (e.g. ecstasy).

Cocaine intoxication presents with all of the features mentioned above, but the effects of cocaine only last between 10 and 30 minutes. Since the patient has presented the following day, cocaine intoxication is unlikely here. Excited delirium is a rare complication of cocaine and other illicit drug intoxication. It is a medical emergency characterised by profuse sweating, delirium, hallucinations, and super human strength. Rhabdomyolysis and hyperkalaemia may follow, leading to cardiac arrest. Discontinuation syndrome is a collection of unpleasant symptoms that occur from suddenly discontinuing an antidepressant. Such symptoms include flu-like symptoms, insomnia, tremors, vertigo, and irritability. This can be prevented by reducing the dose over a 4-week period. Discontinuation syndrome is more common with paroxetine and venlafaxine. Neuroleptic malignant syndrome (NMS) is a rare life-threatening complication of antipsychotics, usually triggered by a new drug or an increase in dose. It presents with rigidity, altered consciousness, and disturbed autonomic function. In severe cases, it may result in rhabdomyolysis, hyperkalaemia, acute kidney failure, and seizures.

17. D

Delirium tremens (DT) is a life-threatening form of alcohol withdrawal which tends to occur 48–96 hours after last exposure to alcohol. It presents with a tremor, hallucinations (classically seeing small people or animals, or feeling insects crawling over their skin), and autonomic dysfunction. Patients may also be delirious or agitated and seizures may occur before the onset of DT. The first-line treatment option for DT is oral lorazepam. It is a medical emergency so patients should be admitted for medically assisted alcohol withdrawal. Benzodiazepines (e.g. lorazepam, diazepam, chlordiazepoxide) are effective at treating psychomotor agitation and mitigating the symptoms of withdrawal. The Clinical Institute Withdrawal Assessment for Alcohol Scale (CIW-Ar) is used to assess the severity of alcohol withdrawal and guide treatment.

Harmful or dependent drinkers should also be offered prophylactic oral thiamine if they are malnourished or at risk of malnourishment, have decompensated liver disease, in acute withdrawal or undergoing medically assisted alcohol withdrawal. Thiamine is important in the prevention of Wernicke's encephalopathy — characterised by ophthalmoplegia, ataxia, and confusion. Chronic thiamine deficiency can also result in Korsakoff syndrome — characterised by anterograde and retrograde amnesia, confabulation, and psychosis. Korsakoff syndrome is irreversible. Alcoholic hallucinosis is a condition in which patients experience hallucinations within 12–24 hours of abstinence, and they typically resolve by 48 hours. Unlike DT, patients will be aware that they are hallucinating and there is no clouding of consciousness or autonomic dysfunction.

18. A

This patient is presenting with several features of schizophrenia (social withdrawal, paranoid delusions, visual hallucinations) and requires prompt treatment. The first-line treatment in the management of schizophrenia is an atypical antipsychotic such as quetiapine, olanzapine, risperidone, amisulpride, and aripiprazole. Although atypical antipsychotics are less likely to cause extra-pyramidal side-effects, they are more strongly associated with causing metabolic changes (including weight gain). As this patient has an eating disorder and has already expressed concern about gaining weight faster than she is comfortable with, it would be appropriate to avoid antipsychotics that are particularly strongly associated with weight gain. Olanzapine and clozapine are strongly associated with weight gain, therefore quetiapine would be the most appropriate option from the listed options.

Mirtazapine is a noradrenergic and specific serotoninergic antidepressant (NaSSA) which is used in the treatment of depression. It has sedative and appetite stimulating effects which helps combat poor sleep and reduced appetite that often accompany depression. Clozapine is used in treatment-resistant schizophrenia. Lithium is a mood stabiliser that is used to treat bipolar disorder.

19. D

Disorders of sexual preference (also known as paraphilias) are abnormalities in sexual practices and desires. They only require treatment if they cause any harm or distress to the patient. Masochism refers to sexual gratification achieved by being humiliated or being in pain.

Sadism is the reverse scenario in which sexual gratification is achieved by inflicting pain on a partner. Fetishism refers to sexual arousal that relies on an inanimate object rather than a person (e.g. leather). Bondage is a sexual practice that involves tying or restraining a sexual partner.

20. C

This patient has presented with features of generalised anxiety disorder (GAD) which is characterised by generalised and persistent anxiety that is not restricted to a particular environment and has lasted for at least 6 months. Patients may complain of autonomic symptoms such as palpitations, sweating, and trembling. The usual first step in the management of GAD involves self-help and psychoeducational groups, however, as this patient has suffered from GAD for a long time and his symptoms are affecting him at work, high-intensity psychological intervention (CBT or applied relaxation), and drug treatment would be more appropriate. The first-line pharmacological treatment for GAD is sertraline (SSRI). If sertraline is unacceptable or ineffective, another SSRI or SNRI could be trialled. If these two classes of drugs are ineffective, pregabalin (a gabapentoid) should be added.

Propranolol is a beta-blocker that is often used to treat the autonomic symptoms of GAD (e.g. palpitations, tremor). It is contraindicated in patients with a past medical history of asthma as it can precipitate bronchoconstriction. Diazepam is a benzodiazepine that has a powerful anxiolytic and sedative effect. As benzodiazepines are addictive, they should only be used for short-term relief of symptoms. Fluoxetine is an SSRI that is not licensed for the treatment of GAD.

The management of GAD is summarised in the following RevChart.

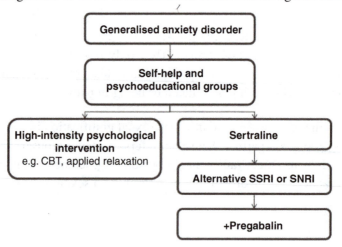

21. A

Post-traumatic stress disorder (PTSD) arises as a delayed response to a stressful event of a catastrophic nature. Symptoms typically need to last longer than 1 month in order to be diagnostic, however, the interval between the event and the onset of symptoms can vary considerably. The main clinical features of PTSD are re-experiencing (e.g. flashbacks, nightmares), avoidance of situations that are reminiscent of the trauma, and autonomic hyperarousal (e.g. hypervigilance, enhanced startle reflex, and insomnia). Other features include emotional blunting, detachment from other people, and anhedonia. Many patients will also describe symptoms of depression and may have suicidal thoughts. Most patients will recover, however, in some patients the disease will follow a chronic course resulting in enduring personality change.

22. D

Lithium has a teratogenic effect in pregnancy and can cause Ebstein's anomaly — a heart malformation in which the tricuspid valve is displaced towards the apex of the heart resulting in atrialisation of the right side of the heart. The risk is particularly high if lithium is used in the first trimester. Decisions regarding the continuation of lithium throughout pregnancy are complex and are dependent on a balance of the risk of relapse of bipolar disorder in pregnancy and the risk of foetal malformations. Some women with bipolar disorder may be switched to an antipsychotic for the duration of the pregnancy.

Several medications can increase the risk of cleft palate including anticonvulsants and methotrexate. Persistent pulmonary hypertension is associated with the use of SSRIs in the third trimester. Spina bifida is usually associated with anticonvulsants, such as sodium valproate and carbamazepine, which are also used as mood stabilisers in the treatment of bipolar disorder. Interrupted aortic arch is a vascular malformation in which there is a gap between the ascending and descending aorta. It is associated with DiGeorge syndrome.

23. C

An overvalued idea is a reasonable idea that is pursued beyond the bounds of reason. In this SBA, thinking that the fence needs redoing is a reasonable idea, however, resigning from work to spend time focusing on this task is unreasonable.

An obsession is a recurrent, unwanted, intrusive thought that enters an individual's mind despite attempts to resist it. It is a defining feature of obsessive compulsive disorder. An obsession may be followed by a compulsion, which is a stereotyped and seemingly purposeful action that the patient feels compelled to carry out despite having an awareness that the thought process is irrational. Mania is a state in which patients experience elevated mood which is out of keeping with the patient's circumstances. Features include overactivity, pressured speech, and reduced need for sleep. A delusion is a fixed belief that is avidly held despite rational argument or evidence to the contrary. It cannot be explained by the patient's cultural, religious or educational background.

24. B

This patient has three features suggestive of opioid overdose: loss of consciousness, pupillary constriction, and respiratory depression. This patient requires urgent IM naloxone which can be given every 2–3 minutes in resuscitation cycles and continued until consciousness is regained and breathing is normal. Naloxone is an opioid antagonist, so beware that this will send the patient into immediate opioid withdrawal. It is not life-threatening, but it can be very distressing as patients experience nausea, fever, abdominal pain, joint and muscle pain, and 'everything runs' (i.e. diarrhoea, vomiting, lacrimation, rhinorrhoea). In contrast to overdose, opioid withdrawal causes pupillary dilatation. This patient will need to be admitted for inpatient monitoring and symptomatic treatment of withdrawal.

Naltrexone is another opioid antagonist; however, it is much slower acting than naloxone so is not effective at treating overdose. It is used to prevent relapse in recovering opioid addicts and alcoholics. Flumazenil is a GABA antagonist used to reverse the effects of benzodiazepine overdose. Whilst these drugs are relatively safe, acute overdose may present with sedation, impaired mental status, respiratory depression, and coma. All psychiatric wards should have a supply of flumazenil as benzodiazepines are often used to sedate agitated patients who may be a danger to themselves or others.

25. D

This patient has experienced an abrupt onset of delusions, hallucinations, and incoherent speech that was precipitated by an acute stressful event. This is suggestive of an acute and transient psychotic disorder. For a diagnosis, the time interval between the first appearance of any psychotic symptoms and the presentation of the fully developed disorder should be less than 2 weeks and there should be no evidence of drug use or organic disease. Full recovery occurs within 3 months (often within days or weeks). It is commonly associated with an acute stressful event (e.g. bereavement), usually preceding the onset of symptoms by 1–2 weeks.

Hallucinations and delusions are first rank symptoms of schizophrenia; however, they must be present for at least one month for schizophrenia to be diagnosed. Furthermore, patients are likely to have other features of schizophrenia such as passivity phenomena, delusional perceptions, and thought alienation. Whilst this patient is exhibiting grandiose delusions and disorganised speech that may suggest a manic episode, there is no elevation in mood, energy or activity. Similarly, depression is unlikely as there is no deterioration in her mood or energy and she is not complaining of any physical symptoms (e.g. insomnia).

Although it is difficult to define what is considered 'normal grief', the Kubler-Ross model outlines the five main stages: denial, anger, bargaining, depression, and acceptance. These stages can occur in a different order and may last varying amounts of time. Features of an abnormal grief reaction include delayed grief occurring more than 2 weeks after the event, and prolonged grief lasting more than 6 months. Pseudo-hallucinations can be part of a normal grieving process and differ from true hallucinations in that the patient has insight that the hallucinations are not real.

26. D

Option A is describing cognitive behavioural therapy (CBT); this is the most widely used talking therapy and it is used to treat depression, anxiety states, PTSD, eating disorders, substance misuse, and insomnia. CBT demonstrates to patients that their thoughts, feelings, and behaviours are all interconnected. For example, a patient with social anxiety may think they will embarrass themselves if they go to a party (thought), this makes them feel worried and stressed (feelings), which prevents them from going to the party (behaviour). This drives a perpetuating cycle of negative thoughts, feelings, and behaviours that worsen the condition and prevent recovery. The aim of CBT is to break this cycle by challenging certain thoughts. For example, a patient with social anxiety could think 'So what if I embarrass myself?' or 'Why do I think I will embarrass myself?'. CBT hopes that an improvement in one component will have a knock-on effect on the other two components. Dialectical behaviour therapy (DBT) is based on the same principles as CBT but has been developed to help patients deal with extreme or unstable emotions; this makes it appropriate for the treatment of emotionally unstable personality disorder. DBT is different from CBT in two main ways: DBT focuses on validation (i.e. teaching the patient how to accept who they are) and the relationship between the therapist and the patient, which is used as motivation to change unhelpful behaviours.

Option E is describing mentalisation-based therapy, which is also used to treat emotionally unstable personality disorder. This therapy is based on the idea that those with BPD have a reduced capacity to mentalise (i.e. think about thinking). The aim of mentalisation-based therapy is to teach patients to recognise and step back from unhelpful thoughts and to assess whether they are valid. Option B is describing eye movement desensitisation and reprocessing (EMDR) which is used to treat PTSD. Patients deliberately recall the trauma in detail whilst fixating on a moving object, which aids memory processing. Option C is describing psychodynamic psychotherapy — this is based on the premise that early childhood experiences have an effect on adult behaviours.

27. B

Bulimia nervosa (BN) is an eating disorder that is characterised by repeated bouts of overeating (bingeing), preoccupation with body weight leading to purging and overconcern about body image. Patients with BN may have a BMI within the normal range because the balance between bingeing and purging may result in little or no change in weight. Dental erosions and caries are common complications of BN resulting from increased exposure to stomach acid and regurgitated carbohydrate-rich fluids. Other complications include irregular or absent periods, swollen salivary glands, cardiac arrhythmias, electrolyte abnormalities (including hyperkalaemia), osteoporosis, and refractory constipation due to excessive laxative abuse. A long history of regurgitation can result in symptoms of gastro-oesophageal reflux disease such as dysphagia and odynophagia, however, it would not affect the motility of the oesophagus. Regular regurgitation could lead to Barrett's oesophagus or, in rare cases, Boerhaave's perforation.

28. C

Clozapine carries a risk of agranulocytosis which can be fatal if not identified and treated early. Therefore, patients on clozapine require a normal leukocyte count before treatment can be initiated and white cell count monitoring weekly for 18 weeks, then every 2 weeks for up to 1 year, and then monthly.

Whilst the typical antipsychotics are associated with extrapyramidal side-effects, the atypical antipsychotics (particularly olanzapine) are associated with hyperprolactinaemia and metabolic complications, such as weight gain, worsening diabetic control, and dyslipidaemia. For all antipsychotic drugs, the following should be monitored:

- Prolactin and fasting blood glucose at baseline, at 6 months and then yearly.
- Blood lipids and weight at baseline, at 3 months and then yearly.
- Patients taking olanzapine or clozapine require more frequent monitoring of these parameters.

Hyponatraemia is associated with all types of antidepressants, particularly SSRIs. Therefore, sodium levels should be checked in any patient on an antidepressant who presents with confusion, drowsiness, or convulsions.

29. E

It is important to discuss potential side-effects whenever a patient is started on any medication. Common side-effects of SSRIs include drowsiness, nausea, dry mouth, insomnia, constipation/diarrhoea, headache, blurred vision, and sexual dysfunction (reduced libido, difficulty reaching orgasm, and erectile dysfunction). Patients may also experience an initial worsening of their anxiety and mood within the first few weeks of starting the medication. Rare side-effects of SSRIs include alopecia, movement disorders, hyponatraemia, and serotonin syndrome.

30. D

Benzodiazepine overdose presents with drowsiness, ataxia, dysarthria, nystagmus, and respiratory depression. The effects of the benzodiazepines need to be reversed with a benzodiazepine antagonist, such as flumazenil. Expert advice needs to be sought before flumazenil can be administered as it can be dangerous in certain patient groups (e.g. patients with benzodiazepine dependence can be pushed into a state of withdrawal). Activated charcoal can be given within one hour of consumption of a poison to reduce absorption in the gastrointestinal tract. It can be used for overdoses of benzodiazepines, aspirin, paracetamol, SSRIs, antipsychotics, and calcium channel blockers. Naloxone is used to reverse opioid overdose and acetylcysteine is used to treat paracetamol overdose. Diazepam is used for cocaine poisoning to reduce agitation. Rapid tranquilisation should be a last resort if verbal de-escalation and other preventative strategies have failed and the patient poses a risk to themselves or others. Patients given rapid tranquilisation need to be monitored every hour to identify any potential complications.

Psychiatry: Paper 2

Questions

1. A 37-year-old truck driver lives by himself and enjoys coin collecting and building model trains. He has never had a sexual partner and has lost touch with his family members. From early childhood, he has never had any close friends and has always preferred to play by himself. He is one of the best truck drivers at his company, but he seems indifferent to praise — he just wants to get the job done and return home to his models. What is the most likely diagnosis?

   A Schizophrenia
   B Depression
   C Schizoid personality disorder
   D Schizotypal personality disorder
   E Emotionally unstable personality disorder

2. A 78-year-old woman is recovering in the surgical ward after having an operation on her shoulder. The operation went well, and she is due for discharge the following day. At 2 am, she is observed pacing around the ward seeming very anxious and complaining about a ringing in her ears. She has a tremor in her hands and is sweating profusely. Which of the following drugs is she likely to be withdrawing from?

  A   Aspirin
  B   Sertraline
  C   Morphine
  D   Temazepam
  E   Paroxetine

3. A 28-year-old man attends the psychiatry outpatient clinic after his
    current treatment has failed to improve his OCD. His obsessions
    are interrupting his life at home as he often has to wake up 3 hours
    before work to check the plug sockets and prepare his clothes.
    It has placed a strain on his relationship with his girlfriend who
    is threatening to leave him. He is currently receiving exposure and
    response prevention therapy and has been on fluoxetine for 4 months
    with no improvement. What is the most appropriate next step in his
    management?

  A   Change to venlafaxine
  B   Change to clomipramine
  C   Change to buspirone
  D   Add quetiapine
  E   Add pregabalin

4. A 25-year-old woman is being reviewed on the psychiatry ward. She
    is detained under section 2 of the mental health act for shop lifting.
    She is visibly distressed, pacing around the room, and snapping at
    the registrar for asking 'idiotic' questions. She says the Mafia are
    after her and the Italian police have planted a chip in her head to
    monitor her thoughts. She screams 'I don't know why I'm telling you
    any of this anyway, you can hear all my thoughts'. What type of delu-
    sion is this patient exhibiting?

  A   Delusional perception
  B   Passivity phenomena
  C   Thought withdrawal
  D   Thought broadcasting
  E   Delusion of reference

5. A worried mother attends the developmental clinic with her 7-year-old son after concerns were raised about his performance at school. His teachers have commented that he finds it difficult to grasp basic concepts. His mother reports that he requires a lot of assistance with daily tasks such as washing and getting dressed. A WISC test is conducted and he is found to have an IQ of 47. What is the most likely diagnosis?

    A Autistic spectrum disorder
    B Attention deficit hyperactivity disorder
    C Mild learning difficulty
    D Moderate learning disability
    E Severe learning disability

6. A 20-year-old woman with an intense fear of gaining weight, purging, and distorted body image is being investigated for anorexia nervosa. Which of the following sets of blood results would you expect to see in this patient?

    A High cortisol, high growth hormone, low cholesterol, low amylase
    B High cortisol, high growth hormone, high cholesterol, low amylase
    C High cortisol, low growth hormone, low cholesterol, high amylase
    D Low cortisol, low growth hormone, high cholesterol, high amylase
    E High cortisol, high growth hormone, high cholesterol, high amylase

7. A 27-year-old man presents to the GP complaining of trouble sleeping. For the last 3 weeks, he has been lying awake for up to 4 hours before falling asleep and has been getting approximately 3 hours of sleep per night. He is worried that this is beginning to affect his career as a carpenter as he has had to cancel jobs due to tiredness. His mood is stable, but he says he has been arguing with his partner due to financial worries. What is the most appropriate management for this patient?

A Give sleep advice only and arrange 2 week follow up
B Give sleep advice and prescribe a short course of temazepam with 2 week follow up
C Give sleep advice and prescribe a short course of diazepam with 2 week follow up
D Refer to a sleep clinic or a specialist with expertise in sleep medicine
E Refer for a cognitive or behavioural intervention

8. A 27-year-old man is referred to the psychiatry clinic after his mother noticed that he has become increasingly socially isolated and his daily functioning has declined over the last year. He has become very impulsive and has been cautioned by the police for public indecency. His speech has become incoherent and he has started making new words which have no apparent meaning. During the consultation, he laughs at unpredictable intervals and answers every question with 'muddy slime and fear'. What is the most likely diagnosis?

A Simple schizophrenia
B Paranoid schizophrenia
C Hebephrenic schizophrenia
D Catatonic schizophrenia
E Undifferentiated schizophrenia

9. A 19-year-old student has been regularly missing his university lectures. He says he feels like the other students are staring at him and gossiping out him. He constantly worries about embarrassing himself and refuses to eat in public. He says that when he enters his lecture hall, he becomes sweaty, feels the urge to urinate and can feel his heart beating. Given the most likely diagnosis, which screening tool would be appropriate to use?

A HADS
B PHQ9
C GAD7
D SADPERSONs scale
E SPIN

10. A 35-year-old man who has recently been diagnosed with schizo-phrenia is started on olanzapine. Within a few days of commencing treatment, he has developed painful contractions of his neck muscles. What is the best treatment option for this condition?

    A Stop olanzapine
    B Reduce olanzapine dose
    C Change to aripiprazole
    D Start tetrabenazine
    E Start procyclidine

11. A 22-year-old woman is reported to the police because of bizarre behaviour. Witnesses say she is dancing naked in the middle of a roundabout and singing lullabies. Police transport her to mental health unit under a section 136. She is incoherent and seems to be talking to someone that is not in the room. She repeats that there are 'people in the walls'. She needs to be detained under the Mental Health Act for further assessment. Which section would be most appropriate in this scenario?

    A Section 2
    B Section 3
    C Section 4
    D Section 17(A)
    E Section 135

12. An 88-year-old woman is being reviewed by the home treatment team. She complains that she does not have the energy to go to the shops anymore and she no longer enjoys watching TV and reading books. She struggles to bring herself to eat three meals per day and has found it difficult to get a full night's sleep. She has a past medical history of an anterior myocardial infarction which occurred 1 year ago. Which of the followings is most appropriate for this patient?

    A Sertraline
    B Fluoxetine
    C Citalopram

    D Clomipramine
    E Venlafaxine

13. A young man with no confirmed identity is being held in A&E under section 136 after he was found wandering alongside a busy motorway. After a few hours of admission, he was able to confirm his identity and appears oriented. It was found that he had walked 40 kms from his home and has no memory of this journey. His memory of events before this incident is intact. What is the most likely diagnosis?

    A Delirium
    B Alzheimer's disease
    C Cannabis-induced psychosis
    D Dissociative fugue
    E Trance and possession disorder

14. A 19-year-old woman presents to A&E in tears after taking a paracetamol overdose. She took 25 paracetamol 500 mg tablets 4 hours ago in an attempt to end her life. She has since realised that this was a mistake and would like to receive treatment. At the time of presentation, she appears well except for some mild nausea. What is the most appropriate next step in her management?

    A Administer activated charcoal
    B Measure plasma paracetamol level
    C Administer IV N-acetylcysteine bolus
    D Start IV N-acetylcysteine infusion
    E Perform gastric lavage

15. A 47-year-old woman with paranoid schizophrenia has had her dose of zuclopenthixol increased to help control delusional symptoms. She is brought into A&E by her son who says she has been drowsy since receiving her zuclopenthixol and feels feverish. On examination, she has a GCS of 11/15 and increased muscle tone in both arms and legs. Her vital signs are shown below:

Heart rate: 132 bpm
Blood pressure: 152/108 mm Hg
Respiratory rate: 18 breaths/min
Temperature: 38.8°C

Given the most likely diagnosis, which blood test is most appropriate?

A Sodium
B Neutrophils
C Prolactin
D Creatine kinase
E Alanine aminotransferase

16. A 12-year-old boy is referred to CAMHS with concerns about his behaviour. He has been caught stealing from the school canteen and has recently been expelled for attempting to start a fire in class. He has had several disciplinary meetings for bullying and fighting. He admits that he does not have friends in school and struggles to concentrate in class. His mother adds that he also misbehaves at home and often starts fights with his 14-year-old brother. His dad is currently in prison for armed robbery and his mum has a history of depression. What is the most likely diagnosis?

A Conduct disorder
B Oppositional defiant disorder
C Depression
D ADHD
E Autism

17. A 26-year-old woman, who was involved in a road traffic accident 6 months ago in which a young man died, has been experiencing regular flashbacks and described feeling constantly on edge whenever she is out of the house. She has avoided travelling in motor vehicles since the accident and has become increasingly socially isolated. As a result, her mood has deteriorated. What is the most appropriate first-line management option?

316 RevMED 300 SBAs in Clinical Specialities

A Trauma-focused CBT
B Exposure and response prevention
C Eye movement desensitisation and reprocessing
D Fluoxetine
E Venlafaxine

18. A distressed 31-year-old man has been referred to the outpatient psychiatry clinic after his behaviour at home changed dramatically. His wife reported that he has been refusing to speak to her and has locked himself in their bedroom several times. When the patient is questioned, he says that he believes that his wife has been replaced by an imposter who is trying to steal his savings. What is the most likely diagnosis?

A Fregoli syndrome
B Capgras syndrome
C De Clerambault syndrome
D Cotard syndrome
E Ekbom syndrome

19. A 43-year-old man has recently been receiving alcohol detoxification treatment from the drugs and alcohol service. He used to drink 750 mL of vodka and 6 cans of beer per day but has since stopped drinking and has just completed a course of chlordiazepoxide as part of assisted withdrawal. He is worried about relapsing and would like to minimise this risk. What is the most appropriate medication to prescribe?

A Diazepam
B Acamprosate
C Naloxone
D Pabrinex
E Disulfiram

20. A 25-year-old man has been admitted to the psychiatry ward under section 2 of the Mental Health Act after he was arrested for

shoplifting and was thought to be acting bizarrely. He claims that he needed a trench coat, sunglasses, and hat to avoid being identified by the secret service. He has supposedly been evading the secret service since he saw a van parked outside his house 6 months ago. He has also maxed out all his credit cards over the last month on elaborate plans to escape surveillance and spends most nights researching methods of making his house invisible to radio signals. He appears dishevelled and his speech is pressured. What is the most likely diagnosis?

    A Mania
    B Schizotypal personality disorder
    C Schizophrenia
    D Shizoaffective disorder
    E Psychotic depression

21. A 26-year-old woman with long-standing depression has attended a family planning clinic. She is currently on paroxetine and would like to know what the risks of continuing her medication during pregnancy would be. Which of the following is associated with SSRI use in pregnancy?

    A Neonatal jaundice
    B Congenital heart disease
    C Spina bifida
    D Systemic hypertension
    E Hydrocephalus

22. A 46-year-old man is brought to see his GP by his wife. She says that he has been acting very strange recently. He used to be very hard-working, getting up at 6 am to start his job as a carpenter, however, he now gets up in the afternoon and doesn't seem to have any interest in his job. He spends most of his time gambling on his laptop. He has also become considerably more aggressive and lashes out physically when challenged on his behaviour. He has been trying to initiate sex more frequently and at inappropriate times. He was involved in a

serious motor cycle accident 6 months ago, which required a prolonged stay in hospital. He appears to have made a full physical
recovery. What is the most likely diagnosis?

    A Manic episode
    B Depressive episode
    C Post-traumatic stress disorder (PTSD)
    D Post-concussion syndrome
    E Frontal lobe syndrome

23. A 25-year-old man is brought into hospital after police found him
rolling around in the street with a mouth full of coins. When asked
where he lives he says, 'I am a superhero, that sandwich is amazing,
my coins are magical'. What kind of thought disorder is this man
exhibiting?

    A Incoherent
    B Circumstantiality
    C Knight's move thinking
    D Tangentiality
    E Flight of ideas

24. A 24-year-old man is brought into A&E by his partner because he has
not slept in over a week. He claims that he does not need to sleep
because his determination to complete his latest project is fueling
him. He claims to be close to creating a new source of renewable
energy that is too complicated for others to understand. He claims
that an angel visits him every night to give him instructions. He
appears agitated and his speech is pressured. What is the most appropriate management option?

    A Start on olanzapine
    B Start on lithium
    C Start on olanzapine and lithium
    D Refer for cognitive behavioural therapy
    E Refer for electroconvulsive therapy

25. A mother brings her 10-year-old son to see his GP to discuss some issues regarding his behaviour. He has been struggling at school and often fails to complete assigned tasks. He is often disruptive in class and fidgets incessantly. His mother has also had difficulty controlling his behaviour at home. The symptoms have been noticeable since he was around 8 years old. What is the most appropriate management option?

    A Watchful waiting
    B Parent training programme
    C Cognitive behavioural therapy
    D Methylphenidate
    E Lisdexamphetamine

26. A 29-year-old woman, who gave birth 6 weeks ago, has been referred to the perinatal mental health clinic after her husband expressed concerns about her behaviour over the last month. She has had trouble bonding with the baby and has been distancing herself from her husband. Furthermore, she is struggling to breastfeed and is feeling inadequate as a mother. What is the most likely diagnosis?

    A Puerperal psychosis
    B Postnatal depression
    C Maternity blues
    D Normal variant
    E Adjustment disorder

27. A 33-year-old heroin user visits his GP with his girlfriend. He has been injecting heroin for 5 years but is intent on stopping and would like some assistance. He has tried to quit once before but experienced severe withdrawal symptoms. What is the most appropriate treatment option?

    A Sublingual buprenorphine
    B IV methadone
    C Oral morphine
    D Oral lofexidine
    E Oral clonidine

28. A 90-year-old lady has just had her fifth fall in 12 months. She is confused and disorientated by her short term memory is intact. She complains that she has seen rats coming out of the wall and climbing over her bed. On examination there is a tremor in the hands. She is on enalapril for hypertension and had a stroke 12 years ago. What is the most likely diagnosis?

    A Vascular dementia
    B Dementia with Lewy bodies
    C Delirium
    D Alzheimer's disease
    E Amnesic syndrome

29. A 65-year-old man with recently diagnosed schizophrenia has been on a course of amisulpride for 6 weeks followed by a course of haloperidol for 6 more weeks with no improvement in symptoms. Both have been trialled at the maximum therapeutic dose. He is still experiencing unpleasant auditory hallucinations and claims that the secret service are spying on him. What is the next best step in his management?

    A Admit for inpatient monitoring
    B Increase the dose of haloperidol
    C Refer for electroconvulsive therapy
    D Start on clozapine
    E Start on olanzapine

30. A 36-year-old woman with treatment-resistant depression is started on lithium to prevent relapses. How does lithium need to be monitored?

    A Lithium levels should be checked weekly after each dose change until a therapeutic level has been achieved and then weekly thereafter
    B Lithium levels should be checked weekly after each dose change until a therapeutic level has been achieved and then monthly thereafter

C Lithium levels should be checked weekly after each dose change until a therapeutic level has been achieved and then 3 monthly thereafter

D Lithium levels should be checked one week after the first dose and then monthly thereafter

E Lithium levels should be checked one week after the first dose and then 3 monthly thereafter

Answers

1. C

Schizoid personality disorder is characterised by disinterest in forming relationships and engaging in sexual relations, indifference to praise, fantasies, and solitary activities. Other features include anhedonia, flat affect, and ignorance of normal social conventions.

Patients with schizotypal personality disorder also have a flat affect and lack close relationships, but they are also likely to be eccentric and have magical or odd beliefs. They may also experience ideas of reference (where real events are misinterpreted as being specific to the patient). Whilst it may appear that this patient could be in the prodromal phase of schizophrenia as he is demonstrating social withdrawal, he is in touch with reality, has behaved like this since childhood and is not exhibiting any first rank symptoms. It is important to remember that both schizotypal and schizoid personality disorders are risk factors for schizophrenia, and some suggest that these three conditions exist on a spectrum. Emotionally unstable personality disorder is associated with intense relationships, self-harm, and chronic feelings of emptiness. Please refer to **Psychiatry: Paper 1, Answers Section, No. 6** for more detail on personality disorders.

2. D

Benzodiazepines, such as diazepam, have a sedative and anxiolytic effect so they are often used in the treatment of insomnia and anxiety states. They are, however, extremely addictive and patients can rapidly develop dependence, so they should only be used in the short term (2–4 weeks). Short-term consequences of benzodiazepine use include drowsiness and reduced consciousness. Prolonged use can result in cognitive impairment, worsening anxiety, and sleep disruption. Features of benzodiazepine withdrawal include insomnia, agitation, anxiety, tremor, tinnitus, and sweating. When withdrawing benzodiazepines, switching patients from short-acting benzodiazepines (e.g. temazepam) to a long-acting benzodiazepine (e.g. diazepam) should be considered, and the dose should be reduced gradually over a number of weeks.

Aspirin does not cause withdrawal symptoms, however, aspirin overdose may cause sweating and tinnitus. Suddenly stopping antidepressants (such as paroxetine and sertraline) can cause discontinuation symptoms such as a flu-like illness and electric shock sensations. Opioid withdrawal may cause dysphoria, nausea, agitation, and diarrhoea.

3. B

The first-line treatment for OCD is a form of CBT called exposure and response prevention (ERP). ERP aims to expose patients to their obsessive thoughts and prevent their compulsions. This restraint will allow anxiety to build, however, patients will eventually habituate and learn to tolerate the anxiety thereby reducing the psychological impact of the obsession. As an adjunct, or if ERP is unsuccessful, an SSRI can be given as they can reduce obsessive thoughts. The preferred SSRI for OCD is fluoxetine, however, others such as paroxetine and sertraline may also be used. Patients should continue SSRI treatment for at least 12 months after remission. If SSRIs are ineffective after 12 weeks of treatment, an alternative SSRI or clomipramine (tricyclic antidepressant) should be trialled.

Venlafaxine is an SNRI used to treat depression. Buspirone is an anxiolytic that is sometimes used in the short-term treatment of GAD. Quetiapine is an atypical antipsychotic that is primarily used to treat psychotic disorders, however, it is occasionally used to augment the treatment of depression and OCD when initial pharmacological therapy is ineffective. Pregabalin is an anti-epileptic that can be used, alongside an antidepressant, in the treatment of GAD.

The management of OCD is summarised in the following RevChart.

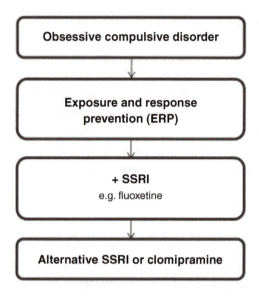

4. D

This patient is demonstrating a delusion called thought alienation — this is a belief that the patient's thoughts are under the control of something or someone else. There are three types of thought alienation: thought withdrawal (thoughts are being removed from the patient's head), thought insertion (thoughts are being placed into the patient's head), and thought broadcasting (thoughts are heard by others). As this patient believes that people can hear her thoughts, it is an example of thought broadcasting. Delusional perception is a two-stage process in which a real perception is interpreted in a delusional way, for example, 'that traffic light turned red, so aliens will invade tomorrow'. Passivity phenomena is the belief that a patient is being controlled by an external power. This can include control of actions, feelings, and impulses. Thought alienation, passivity phenomena, and delusional perception are components of Schneider's first rank symptoms of schizophrenia, along with auditory hallucinations. First rank symptoms are suggestive of schizophrenia in the absence of organic disease but are not necessary to make the diagnosis as they can occur in mania and delirium and are absent in 20% of patients with schizophrenia.

A delusion of reference is the belief that events, or actions of others have a special significance for the patient. For example, believing that the news correspondent on TV is trying to convey a secret message to the patient. Delusions of reference are seen in schizophrenia, bipolar disorder, and delusional disorder.

5. D

It is important to make a clear distinction between a learning difficulty and a learning disability. A learning disability is characterised by a limitation in intellectual functioning, maladaptive behaviour across several environments which is apparent from childhood, and an IQ below 70. It can be further classified based on IQ as follows:

- 50–70: Mild
- 35–49: Moderate
- 20–34: Severe
- Less than 20: Profound

Therefore, the child in this question has a moderate learning disability. A learning *difficulty* is a condition in which general intelligence is unaffected, but the patient has some difficulties processing a specific type of information (e.g. dyslexia, dyspraxia). There are several age-specific IQ tests which are used in different paediatric populations including the Wechsler Preschool and Primary Scale of Intelligence (WPPSI) designed for children aged 2–7 years, and the Wechsler Intelligence Scale for Children (WISC) which is designed for children aged 6–16 years.

Autistic spectrum disorder typically presents with a triad of difficulties with reciprocal social interaction, difficulties with communication, and the presence of restricted, repetitive behaviour. It typically presents before the age of 3 years. Attention deficit hyperactivity disorder (ADHD) presents with features of hyperactivity and inattention which must occur in more than one environment and must be present for over 6 months.

6. E

Cortisol is a stress hormone that is increased in anorexia nervosa to stimu-late gluconeogenesis and maintain a sufficiently high blood glucose level whilst the body is in a state of starvation. Similarly, growth hormone secretion is increased in response to fasting and it also helps stimulate gluconeogenesis, lipolysis, and protein synthesis. The mechanism that causes hypercholesterolaemia in anorexia nervosa is not fully understood but it may be due to increased cholesterol ester transfer protein activity. Amylase, produced by the parotid glands, is also elevated after repeated bouts of purging. Other important laboratory findings in anorexia nervosa are listed in the following table.

Blood test	Result
FBC	Low Hb, WCC, platelets
U&E	Low urea, hyponatraemia, hypokalaemia
Phosphate	Low
LFTs	ALP and bilirubin high
CK	High
Glucose	Low
TFTs	T3 low, TSH high (hypothyroid)
FSH, LH, oestrogen, progesterone	Low
Calcium, magnesium	Low
Amylase	High
Chloride	Low
Cortisol, GH	High
Cholesterol	High

7. B

Insomnia encompasses difficulty getting to sleep, difficulty staying asleep, or inadequate sleep resulting in impaired daytime functioning. Insomnia can be classified in two ways: primary (when no comorbidity is identified) and secondary (occurring as a result of another condition), or short-term (<4 weeks) and long-term (>4 weeks). The duration of insomnia determines the course of management. Short-term insomnia is managed with sleep hygiene advice (e.g. relaxing before bed, maintaining a comfortable sleeping environment, avoiding daytime napping, avoiding caffeine, nicotine, and alcohol). If there is severe daytime impairment (as in this case), a short course of a hypnotic agent may be considered. The hypnotics that are recommended are short-acting benzodiazepines (e.g. temazepam) and non-benzodiazepine 'Z-drugs' (e.g. zopiclone). Diazepam can be used if insomnia is associated with daytime anxiety. If a hypnotic is prescribed, the lowest possible dose should be used for the shortest possible time, and the patient should be reviewed after 2 weeks.

For long-term insomnia, sleep hygiene should be reviewed and whilst pharmacological therapy is not recommended, a hypnotic drug can be used for up to 4 weeks. These medications can cause dependency and withdrawal with prolonged use. In people over the age of 55 years, modified-release melatonin may be considered, and this can be used for up to 13 weeks. These patients can also be referred for a cognitive or behavioural intervention (e.g. CBT, relaxation training, sleep restriction therapy, and stimulus control therapy). If primary care fails to manage the insomnia, the patient can be referred to a sleep clinic or a specialist with expertise in sleep medicine.

8. C

Schizophrenia is a psychotic disorder characterised by distortions in thinking and perception, inappropriate or blunted affect with clear consciousness. It often features Schneider's first rank symptoms (see **Psychiatry: Paper 2, Answers Section, No. 4**). There are several subtypes of schizophrenia which are defined based on the combination of prominent features present. Hebephrenic schizophrenia (also known as disorganised schizophrenia) is characterised by affective changes (usually shallow or inappropriate), disorganised thought and speech, fleeting delusions, and irresponsible behaviour. Patients may sometimes be described as having a 'childlike' demeanour. It is usually diagnosed in adolescents and young adults and tends to have a poor prognosis due to the rapid development of negative symptoms.

Paranoid schizophrenia is the most common subtype of schizophrenia. It is dominated by stable, paranoid delusions that are usually accompanied by pronounced hallucinations. Catatonic schizophrenia features prominent psychomotor disturbances that can range from hyperkinesis to stupor. Other manifestations include automatic obedience (with motor tasks) and negativism (resisting being moved). Simple schizophrenia refers to the gradual development of abnormal behaviour that results in a decline in day-to-day functioning. The negative features of schizophrenia tend to be prominent without any psychotic symptoms. Undifferentiated schizophrenia is a broad term used to describe psychotic conditions that meet the diagnostic criteria for schizophrenia but do not fit into any specific subtype.

9. E

Social phobia is a relatively common condition in which patients have an intense fear of being scrutinised by others and embarrassing themselves. This can manifest with physical symptoms, similar to panic attacks, when entering social situations. There are two screening tools that can be used to assess the severity of social phobia: social phobia inventory (SPIN) and the Liebowitz social anxiety scale. Other screening tools used in psychiatry include the hospital anxiety and depression scale (HADS), patient health questionnaire 9 (PHQ9) for depression, generalised anxiety disorder 7 (GAD 7), and the SADPERSONs scale which is used to assess suicide risk.

10. E

Acute dystonia is an extra-pyramidal side-effect of antipsychotic medications. It is characterised by the development of involuntary, sustained, painful muscle contractions. They may affect the neck, causing torticollis. Other extra-pyramidal side-effects include Parkinsonism, tardive dyskinesia, and akathisia. Extra-pyramidal side-effects can be caused by any antipsychotic medication, however, they are more common with typical antipsychotics. Acute dystonia usually starts soon after commencing antipsychotic medication and should be treated with procyclidine (an anticholinergic).

Features of drug-induced Parkinsonism include a resting tremor, rigidity, and bradykinesia. Akathisia is a persistent feeling of restlessness which can be treated by reducing the dose of antipsychotic or by giving propranolol or low-dose clonazepam. Tardive dyskinesia causes involuntary, writhing body movements including grimacing and sticking the tongue out. They usually develop in patients with a history of long-term antipsychotic use and can be treated using tetrabenazine. It is important to differentiate between acute dystonia and tardive dyskinesia as anticholinergics, like procyclidine, can make tardive dyskinesia worse.

11. A

This patient is acutely psychotic and is posing a serious risk to herself. She therefore requires urgent assessment and treatment. The most appropriate section is a section 2 as this allows a 28-day period for the patient to be assessed and treated. This section may be extended to a section 3 if it is thought that the patient needs to remain in hospital to receive treatment. For more information regarding the different types of section, please refer to the table on **Psychiatry: Paper 1, Answers Section, No. 11**.

12. A

The major classes of antidepressant drugs include the selective serotonin reuptake inhibitors (SSRIs, e.g. sertraline), tricyclic antidepressants (TCAs, e.g. clomipramine), serotonin and noradrenaline reuptake inhibitors (SNRIs, e.g. venlafaxine), and monoamine oxidase inhibitors. There is relatively little difference between the classes of drugs in terms of efficacy, so the choice is often based on patient factors, such as pre-existing disease, current therapies, suicide risk, and previous response to antidepressants. SSRIs are better tolerated and are safer in overdose than other classes and are therefore, considered first line for depression. Sertraline, fluoxetine, and citalopram are all SSRIs that can be used in depression, but the most appropriate choice, in this scenario, is sertraline as it is safest in patients with a history of ischaemic heart disease. TCAs are used more sparingly than SSRIs because they are cardiotoxic and have anticholinergic (e.g. dry mouth, drowsiness, blurred vision, urinary retention) and antihistaminic (e.g. weight gain, sedation) side-effects.

Side-effects associated with SSRIs and SNRIs are similar and typically include gastrointestinal upset (e.g. diarrhoea, constipation, abdominal pain, loss of appetite), insomnia, loss of libido, and sexual dysfunction. All patients starting antidepressants should be warned that there is a risk of experiencing increased anxiety and depression in the first few weeks of treatment, and that it often takes 4–6 weeks for the effects to become apparent.

13. D

A dissociative disorder (also known as conversion disorder) is when a patient experiences loss of the integration between memories of the past, awareness of identity, and immediate sensations and control of bodily movements. They are often linked to traumatic events. This SBA describes dissociative fugue which is a subtype of dissociative disorder characterised by amnesia and purposeful travel beyond the usual everyday range. Despite the amnesia experienced during the episode, the patient's behaviour during this period may appear normal to an independent observer. An important distinction to make is that only disorders of physical functions under voluntary control and loss of sensation fall under dissociative disorders, whereas disorder involving pain and the autonomic nervous system are classified as somatisation disorders. All types of dissociative disorders tend to remit after a few weeks or months.

Trance and possession disorder is a type of dissociative disorder which causes temporary loss of personal identity with full awareness of the surroundings. Delirium is an acute confusional state resulting from an underlying physical cause. It leads to clouding of consciousness and can cause memory loss. Alzheimer's disease causes anterograde amnesia and has a more chronic course that does not remit. Cannabis-induced psychosis is more likely to present with psychotic symptoms.

14. B

Paracetamol overdose is a common mode of attempted suicide. An overdose of paracetamol saturates the ability of the liver to metabolise paracetamol resulting in the accumulation of a toxic intermediate called N-acetyl-p-benzoquinone imine (NAPQI) which is hepatotoxic and can cause fulminant liver failure. Patients may be asymptomatic or have non-specific symptoms such as nausea for the first 24 hours. Thereafter, they will become severely unwell with severe abdominal pain. During this phase, prothrombin time and transaminases will be raised. The management of paracetamol overdose first involves measuring the plasma paracetamol level at 4 hours after ingestion. This value will be plotted on a normogram which helps determine whether treatment with an IV N-acetylcysteine infusion is necessary.

If patients are presenting within 2 hours of ingestion, treatment with activated charcoal can be considered as it reduces absorption of paracetamol. Gastric lavage is another method of preventing paracetamol absorption, however, it is not routinely performed.

15. D

Neuroleptic malignant syndrome (NMS) is a complication of taking antipsychotic drugs that presents with muscle rigidity, fever, altered consciousness, and disturbed autonomic function. Elevated serum creatine kinase (CK) is the most specific blood abnormality associated with NMS. The degree of CK elevation correlates with severity and prognosis.

Whilst leucocytosis, transaminitis, and electrolyte abnormalities commonly occur in NMS, these are non-specific changes and can have multiple causes. Complications of NMS include acute renal failure associated with rhabdomyolysis, seizures, cardiac arrhythmias, and disseminated intravascular coagulation. The causative agent needs to be stopped immediately and treatment is mainly supportive (e.g. fluids, cooling blankets, DVT prophylaxis). Some specific medical therapies include lorazepam for agitation, dantrolene (muscle relaxant) for malignant hyperthermia, and bromocriptine to reverse the dopamine blockade. Hyperprolactinaemia is also associated with antipsychotics, but this presents with galactorrhoea, amenorrhoea, gynaecomastia, and sexual dysfunction.

16. A

Conduct disorder (CD) is defined as a repetitive and persistent pattern of behaviour in which the basic rights of others are violated. CD manifests with behaviours belonging to four subgroups: aggression to people and animals (e.g. bullying, fighting, cruelty to animals, sexual assault), destruction of property (e.g. fire-setting, vandalism), deceitfulness or theft (e.g. shoplifting, breaking, and entering), and serious violations of rules (e.g. truancy, staying out late). For a diagnosis of CD, at least three of these features have to be present for at least 12 months and the behaviour must impair social, academic, or occupational functioning. Risk factors include a family history of mental health conditions, urban upbringing, low socio-economic class, harsh and inconsistent parenting, and parental substance abuse. CD is one of the most common reasons for referrals to CAMHS.

Oppositional defiant disorder is a milder type of CD that occurs in children under 11 years old and is characterised by arguing with and disobeying adults without the extreme behaviours present in CD. Children with conduct disorders often have other mental health problems, particularly attention deficit hyperactivity disorder (ADHD). For a diagnosis of ADHD, at least six symptoms of inattention and hyperactivity must occur before the age of 12 years, be present in two or more settings and interfere with social, educational, or occupational function. Whilst this child does display some features of inattention present in ADHD, there are no features of hyperactivity. Depression may rarely present with antisocial behaviour in children but is more likely to present with classical features of depression (e.g. anergia, anhedonia). Autism is another important diagnosis to consider. Although this patient does show evidence of impaired social interaction, there is no delay in speech and language, and no evidence of repetitive, ritualistic behaviours.

17. A

This patient has developed post-traumatic stress disorder (PTSD) which is a delayed response to a stressful situation of an exceptionally threatening nature. It is characterised by re-experiencing the event (e.g. nightmares, flashbacks), avoidance of activities reminiscent of the event, and autonomic hyperarousal (e.g. exaggerated startle reflex). Patients may develop depression and suicidal thoughts. The first-line treatment option for PTSD is trauma-focused CBT, which examines the thought processes that have been shaped by the traumatic event and attempts to restructure these belief systems.

Eye movement desensitisation and reprocessing (EMDR) is another form of psychological therapy that is used in PTSD. Patients deliberately narrate the event whilst fixing their eyes on the therapist's finger as it passes from side to side. This aids memory processing. Exposure and response prevention is a psychological treatment that is used to treat OCD. Although they are not routinely recommended, antidepressants can be used in the treatment of PTSD. The most commonly used in the treatment of PTSD are sertraline, paroxetine, venlafaxine, or mirtazapine.

18. B

Capgras syndrome is a delusional disorder in which the patient believes that someone they associate closely with (such as a spouse) has been replaced by an imposter. This delusion typically occurs in patients with schizophrenia.

Fregoli syndrome is a similar delusional disorder in which the patient believes that different people are, in fact, a single shape-shifting individual who is intent on persecuting the patient. De Clerambault syndrome, also known as erotomania, is a delusional disorder in which the patient that someone (who they may never have met) is madly in love with them. Patients may also experience delusions of reference where they believe that their admirer is sending secret messages to them. Cotard syndrome is a delusion that occurs in severely depressed patients where they believe that they are dead or that their body parts are rotting. Ekbom syndrome, also known as delusional parasitosis, is characterised by the delusional belief that the patient has been parasitised by insects. Patients may complain of a sensation of insects crawling under their skin (formication).

19. B

Assisted withdrawal from alcohol dependence typically involves giving a reducing dose of a benzodiazepine (such as chlordiazepoxide or diazepam) over 7–10 days. This allows the alcohol to exit the patient's body whilst the benzodiazepines ameliorate the symptoms of withdrawal. Once assisted withdrawal has been completed, some patients may request treatment to reduce the risk of relapse. The first-line treatment for the prevention of relapse are acamprosate and naltrexone, which have an anti-craving effect. These medications work best alongside individualised psychological intervention.

Disulfiram, an acetaldehyde dehydrogenase inhibitor, is another drug that can be used for prevention of relapse as it makes patients experience symptoms of a hangover immediately after drinking alcohol. However, it tends to be used as a second-line option if acamprosate and naltrexone are unsuccessful or unacceptable. Diazepam can be used as an alternative to chlordiazepoxide for assisted withdrawal, however, as they are addictive, they should not be used long-term. Naloxone is a μ-opioid receptor antagonist commonly used to treat opioid overdose. Pabrinex is a solution containing several vitamins which is used to prevent Wernicke–Korsakoff syndrome in alcoholics.

20. D

Schizoaffective disorder is a condition in which both psychotic and affective symptoms are present to the same extent. There are two main types of schizoaffective disorder: manic and depressive. This patient has manic features (pressured speech, excessive spending, lack of sleep) on a background of a psychotic delusion that preceded the mania. An important distinction to make is that in schizoaffective disorder the psychotic symptoms are present irrespective of their affective state, whereas in mania with psychosis or psychotic depression the psychotic symptoms occur when their mood symptoms are most severe, and delusions tend to be mood congruent.

Schizophrenia presents with positive symptoms (hallucinations, delusions) and negative symptoms (social withdrawal, lack of function) but typically causes a blunted affect as opposed to depression or mania.

Schizotypal personality disorder is characterised by eccentric behaviour, bizarre ideas, cold affect, and a tendency to social withdrawal. It resembles schizophrenia but the symptoms are not prominent enough to reach a diagnosis of schizophrenia.

21. B

SSRI use in pregnancy is associated with an increased risk of congenital heart disease (if used in the first trimester) and an increased risk of persistent pulmonary hypertension (if used in the third trimester). Decisions about using SSRIs in pregnancy are based on the severity of the depression and weighing up the risks and benefits. Paroxetine, in particular, is associated with an increased risk of congenital malformations. SSRIs that are generally considered safer in pregnancy include sertraline, citalopram, and fluoxetine, so this patient may be offered a change in her medication. Paroxetine and sertraline are considered safe to use during breastfeeding.

22. E

This patient is displaying features suggestive of frontal lobe syndrome — executive dysfunction (e.g. poor judgement, problem-solving, and decision-making), change in social behaviour and personality (e.g. sexual disinhibition, impulsivity, lability), and apathy (e.g. lack of motivation). Other features of frontal lobe syndrome include a lack of insight into the personality change, forced utilisation (where patients use objects in an appropriate way but at an inappropriate time, for example, seeing a bed and then getting into bed during the middle of day), and re-emergence of primitive reflexes. Frontal lobe syndrome is caused by head injury, stroke, tumours, Alzheimer's disease, and frontotemporal dementia. In this case, it is likely to be linked to the motorcycle accident. Frontotemporal dementia (Pick's disease) is an umbrella term for six types of dementia involving the frontal and/or temporal lobes, which can cause a frontal lobe syndrome. It causes frontotemporal atrophy due to the accumulation of Tau bodies.

An affective disorder should certainly be explored in this patient as he is showing signs of mania (e.g. increased libido, gambling, aggression, and sexual disinhibition) and depression (e.g. no longer enjoying things he used to enjoy). However, with mania, one would expect an elevation in mood and energy, with increased confidence or grandiose thoughts. The opposite would be expected with depression — features include physical symptoms (e.g. decreased sleep, appetite, concentration, and libido) and thoughts of guilt, worthlessness, and self-harm. PTSD is a plausible option given the patient's recent road traffic accident. However, PTSD is unlikely as this patient has not complained of flashbacks, nightmares, avoidance, and hyperarousal. Post-concussion syndrome is a set of symptoms that may persist for weeks to months following a concussion. Symptoms tend to be psychological (e.g. depression, anxiety, poor concentration, and memory), but physical symptoms may occur (e.g. headaches, dizziness, insomnia).

23. C

Knight's move thinking (derailment) is a thought disorder characterised by unexpected and illogical leaps between ideas without apparent connections. It is most commonly found in schizophrenia and acute psychotic states.

Flight of ideas is accelerated speech with abrupt changes in topic that is seemingly lacking purpose. Unlike Knight's move thinking, there may be discernible connections between ideas, and these are usually based around understandable associations, distractions (e.g. something the patient sees or hears) and plays on words (e.g. clang associations). Flight of ideas is a feature of mania. Circumstantiality is when patients provide excessive, unnecessary detail about a story before eventually returning to the original point. Tangentiality is when patients wander off a topic when answering a question, and never return to answering the question. Incoherence or word salad is when real words are strung together into nonsensical sentences.

24. A

The diagnostic criteria for a manic episode are as follows:

- A period of persistently elevated, expansive or irritable mood, lasting at least 1 week.

- During this period, at least three of the following may be present: increased self-esteem, decreased sleep, more talkative or pressure to talk, flight of ideas, distractibility, increase in goal-directed activity or psychomotor agitation and excessive involvement in risky behaviours (e.g. gambling, unsafe sex).
- The symptoms do not meet criteria for bipolar affective disorder.
- The symptoms are severe enough to impair occupational or social functioning.
- The symptoms are not due to the direct effects of a substance (e.g. illicit drugs) or a medical condition (e.g. hyperthyroidism).

Acute manic episodes are managed with antipsychotic drugs (olanzapine, quetiapine, or risperidone). If the response is inadequate, lithium or valproate may be added. Four weeks after the acute episode has resolved, lithium is the first-line option for the prevention of relapse. However, if lithium is poorly tolerated or the response is inadequate, olanzapine or valproate can be given alone or as an adjunct with lithium. Cognitive behavioural therapy can also be used alongside lithium to prevent relapses of manic episodes. Electroconvulsive therapy (ECT) involves sending an electric current through the brain under general anaesthesia to produce a generalised tonic–clonic seizure. It is only recommended in severe acute mania that is unresponsive to medical treatment.

25. B

Attention deficit hyperactivity disorder (ADHD) is characterised by features of inattention and hyperactivity lasting more than 6 months in more than one situation (e.g. school and home). It typically presents in children who are aged 6–12 years. The first-line treatment option for ADHD is an ADHD-focused group parent training programme. This involves educating parents about ADHD and parenting strategies. If parent training is unsuccessful or unacceptable, medication may be considered. The first-line pharmacological treatment is methylphenidate (also known by its brand name, Ritalin). Other pharmacological options include lisdexamphetamine, dexamphetamine, and atomoxetine. An important complication of pharmacological treatment is reduced appetite and growth, so it is important to monitor the patient's height and weight when receiving treatment. If, unlike in this SBA, the patient has symptoms suggestive of ADHD but not meeting the full criteria, a 10-week watch and wait period should be completed before treatment is considered.

26. B

Postnatal depression is a form of depression that around 10% of women experience soon after giving birth. It can occur at any time within 1 year of giving birth. It presents in much the same way as depression with core symptoms of low mood, anhedonia, and anergia. Patients may also complain of difficulty bonding with the baby, withdrawing from social contacts and, in severe cases, thoughts of hurting the baby. The severity can be assessed using the Edinburgh Postnatal Depression scale. Postnatal depression can be treated with cognitive behavioural therapy or antidepressants. Although antidepressants can be secreted in breastmilk, they are recommended if the benefits outweigh the risks. The safest antidepressants to use when breastfeeding are sertraline and paroxetine. In severe cases with suicidal or infanticidal ideation, admission to a mother and baby unit should be considered. Prompt treatment of postnatal depression is important to prevent issues with the baby's attachment which can have lasting effects on their development.

Maternity blues, also known as baby blues, is a common condition occurring within 2 weeks of childbirth. It is characterised by emotional lability, low mood, tearfulness, and anxiety. Patients often recover promptly. In the presence of prolonged symptoms, a diagnosis of postnatal depression should be considered. Puerperal psychosis is a mental health disorder that typically manifests from around 2 weeks after childbirth. Patients present with features of psychotic depression, mania, or psychosis. Symptoms fluctuate and most patients recover within 6–12 weeks.

27. A

The mainstay for assisted withdrawal from heroin is to use a substitute such as methadone or buprenorphine. Methadone is a μ-opioid receptor agonist that has a long half-life and causes a less intense high, thereby ameliorating the withdrawal effects as patients come off heroin. Methadone is usually given as an oral liquid (not IV). Buprenorphine is a partial agonist of the μ-opioid receptor and can be given in a sublingual preparation during detoxification treatment.

Oral morphine is not used as a substitute for heroin during detoxification. Lofexidine and clonidine are α_2 agonists that may be considered if substitution with methadone or buprenorphine are unacceptable or if dependence is mild. They may help reduce some of the symptoms of opioid withdrawal (e.g. agitation, anxiety). Other symptomatic treatments used to manage some of the manifestations of opioid withdrawal include anti-diarrhoeals, anti-emetics, and analgesics. Patients undergoing detoxification should also have a key worker appointed, who will support the patient throughout the process. Screening for blood-borne infections would also be a sensible measure in a patient with a history of IV drug use.

28. B

This patient is exhibiting the classical triad of Dementia with Lewy Bodies (DLB): confusion, vivid visual hallucinations, and Parkinsonian signs (e.g. tremor). Parkinsonism is a late sign and may also include rigidity, bradykinesia, and postural instability. DLB is a progressive disease caused by the accumulation of alpha synuclein proteins (Lewy bodies) in neurons, resulting in their degradation. Whilst this patient does have significant vascular risk factors, the history does not suggest an acute and step-wise deterioration in cognitive function that is characteristic of vascular dementia. Alzheimer's disease is also unlikely as it is characterised by an eroded personality and a loss of short-term memory. Refer to the following table for more key differences between these three subtypes of dementia.

	Alzheimer's disease	Vascular dementia	Dementia with Lewy bodies
Risk factors	Age, vascular risk factors, low IQ/ poorly educated, head injury, family history	Age, vascular risk factors	Age, largely unknown

(Continued)

(Continued)

	Alzheimer's disease	Vascular dementia	Dementia with Lewy bodies
Histopathology	Atrophy, plaque formation, NFTs, cholinergic neuronal loss	Multiple cortical infarcts, arteriosclerosis	Lewy bodies
Onset	Insidious	Sudden	Varies
Course	Gradual decline	Stepwise decline	Gradual decline
Main features	Amnesia, apraxia, agnosia, aphasia	Patchy cognitive impairment	Fluctuating confusion, visual hallucinations, Parkinsonian symptoms
Affect	Depression or anxiety (early), flattened affect (later)	Depression, lability	Depression
Other features	Absence of physical signs	Focal neurology	Repeated falls, syncope, transient losses of consciousness, neuroleptic sensitivity
Personality	Eroded: *'it's just not mum anymore'*, social withdrawal	Relatively preserved	More apathetic
CT changes	Generalised atrophy, especially temporal and parietal	Multiple lucencies	Mild atrophy

Delirious patients may develop hallucinations and delusions, but delirium tends to have a relatively rapid onset, lasts for less than 6 months and patients' consciousness will be impaired. Amnesic syndrome is characterised by anterograde and retrograde memory loss (i.e. the patient is unable to form new memories and pre-existing memories are lost). The most common cause is Korsakoff syndrome, which is caused by severe thiamine deficiency. These patients characteristically confabulate and retain procedural memory.

29. D

This patient has treatment-resistant schizophrenia — defined as failure to respond to two or more antipsychotics, at least one of which is an atypical agent, each given at a therapeutic dose for at least 6 weeks. Clozapine is the first-line option for treatment-resistant schizophrenia. Clozapine carries several potentially fatal complications, such as agranulocytosis. A normal leucocyte count is necessary before treatment can be initiated and then a full blood count should be checked weekly for 18 weeks, then every 2 weeks for up to 1 year and then monthly. Other complications include myocarditis and cardiomyopathy, neuroleptic malignant syndrome, and impairment of intestinal peristalsis (including constipation, obstruction, and ileus).

It may be necessary to consider admitting this patient to a psychiatric ward to initiate the treatment if he is deemed to be a risk to himself or others, but this is not absolutely necessary. Haloperidol has already been attempted at a therapeutic dose without success, and therefore, increasing the dose would only increase the risk of side-effects. Electroconvulsive therapy is used in treatment-resistant depression, mania, and catatonic schizophrenia. Olanzapine is an atypical agent and is inappropriate in this situation as amisulpride has already been trialled without success.

30. C

Lithium requires careful monitoring because it has a narrow therapeutic range (0.4–1 mmol/l). Routine serum lithium monitoring should be performed weekly after initiation and after each dose change until a therapeutic level has been achieved. It should then be checked every 3 months thereafter. Additional measurements are required if there is a significant change in the patient's sodium or fluid intake. Before initiation of lithium, renal function (U&Es), cardiac function (ECG) and thyroid function (TFTs) and FBC should be requested, and BMI should be measured. BMI, renal function, and thyroid function should also be monitored every 6 months during treatment.

Lithium has an extensive side-effect profile which can be remembered using the mnemonic **LITHIUM**:

- **L**eucocytosis
- **I**nsipidus (nephrogenic)
- **T**remor
- **H**ypothyroidism
- **I**ncreased **u**rine output
- **M**others (teratogenic)
- **O**ther: gastrointestinal upset, weight gain, and T-wave inversion

A life-threatening complication of lithium therapy is lithium toxicity, which usually occurs when the plasma concentration exceeds 1.2 mmol/L. This most often occurs due to reduced excretion of the drug caused by dehydration, reduced renal function, infections, and drugs that interfere with lithium excretion (e.g. NSAIDs and diuretics). Deliberate overdoses are a rarer cause. Lithium toxicity presents with vomiting, diarrhoea, ataxia, weakness, dysarthria, and tremor. Plasma lithium concentrations exceeding 2 mmol/L are associated with convulsions, renal failure, and coma. Lithium should be stopped immediately, and supportive treatment should be commenced. Gastric lavage may be considered if it can be performed within an hour of an overdose.

Index

infertility, 225
inflammatory bowel disease (IBD), 55, 123
influenza vaccine, 28
inheritance pattern, 21
innocent murmurs, 63
insomnia, 326
instrumental delivery, 199
intestinal malrotation, 98
intracytoplasmic sperm injection (ICSI), 151
intrauterine device (IUD), 259
intrauterine growth restriction (IUGR), 264
intrauterine insemination (IUI), 151
intrauterine system, 259
intussusception, 12, 80
in vitro fertilisation (IVF), 151
iron deficiency anaemia, 200
irritable bowel syndrome, 125
irritant dermatitis, 134

J
juvenile idiopathic arthritis (JIA), 45, 58, 79

K
Kallmann syndrome, 28
Kawasaki disease, 59, 79
kernicterus, 133
Kleihauer test, 269
Korsakoff syndrome, 300
Krukenberg tumour, 187
Kubler-Ross model, 305

L
labetalol, 151
labial fusion, 57

lactational amenorrhoea, 266
lactational mastitis, 186
large loop excision of the transformation zone (LLETZ), 202, 256
laryngomalacia, 94
learning difficulty, 325
learning disability, 325
lichen sclerosus, 260
linea nigra, 229
lithium, 301, 303, 341
lochia, 197
lorazepam, 300
low-lying placenta, 261
lymphoma, 31

M
(MMR) vaccine, 255
macrocephaly, 119
magnesium sulphate, 224
malingering, 297
mania, 336
Marfan syndrome, 21
maternity blues, 338
McRoberts manouevre, 229
measles, 89
Meckel's diverticulum, 80, 125
meconium aspiration, 24
Meigs syndrome, 187
memantine, 299
meningitis, 20, 120
meningococcal sepsis, 90
menopause, 203, 238
Mental Health Act, 294
mentalisation-based therapy, 306
mesenteric adenitis, 55
microcephaly, 120
mid-luteal progesterone, 155